Essential Skills for Managing in Healthcare

Essential Skills for Managing in Healthcare

ANDREW PRICE

Leadership Development Consultant

and

ANDREW SCOWCROFT

Managing Director
Development Consultancy, Cardiff

Foreword by

JOHN EDMONSTONE

Director, MTDS Consultancy
Senior Research Fellow
School of Public Policy and Professional Practice
University of Keele

Radcliffe Publishing
Oxford • New York

Radcliffe Publishing Ltd
18 Marcham Road
Abingdon
Oxon OX14 1AA
United Kingdom

www.radcliffepublishing.com

Electronic catalogue and worldwide online ordering facility.

British Library Cataloguing in Publication Data

A catalogue record for this book is available from the British Library.

ISBN-13: 978 184619 480 1

The paper used for the text pages of this book is FSC certified. FSC (The Forest Stewardship Council) is an international network to promote responsible management of the world's forests.

Mixed Sources
Product group from well-managed forests and other controlled sources
www.fsc.org Cert no. SGS-COC-2482
© 1996 Forest Stewardship Council

FSC

Typeset by Pindar NZ, Auckland, New Zealand
Printed and bound by TJI Digital, Padstow, Cornwall, UK

Contents

Foreword

We live in an era in which it has become clearer and clearer what good leadership and managerial practice at work is. We know that if we are to attract and retain excellent staff and get them to 'go the extra mile' then we have to treat them with respect, empathy and skill, and that the quality of our relationships with them is a major key to success. Yet report after report, survey after survey, show that many staff feel undervalued by their leaders and managers, whom they typically describe as 'arrogant', 'insensitive' and 'clumsy'. As one employee told me in a focus group looking at employee engagement, 'They regard us as human doings, not human beings!'

Clearly no one does this deliberately and many leaders and managers would be amazed and incredulous if they were able to hear what their staff really felt. Andrew Scowcroft and Andrew Price suggest that we should begin with an expectation that people will be led and managed well at work and that this should be the norm and not a lucky bonus. As they point out, no one would expect such professionals as doctors and lawyers to learn on the job, but that this is usually the case with leaders and managers. This book is dedicated to helping leaders and managers prepare for those responsibilities by focusing on working with individuals, teams and change. It also addresses three areas that usually make leaders and managers uncomfortable – running meetings successfully, making presentations and writing reports. Getting all these aspects right will go a long way towards ensuring that instead of negative reports, we will begin to hear staff say that they are 'pleasantly surprised' and even 'delighted' by the way that they are treated.

Making (and mending) working relationships is *the* means of building up the social capital that our organisations increasingly rely on to succeed in this interdependent world. This book gives accessible and practical examples of how this can be done and I have no hesitation in commending it to a wide readership.

John Edmonstone
Director, MTDS Consultancy
Senior Research Fellow
School of Public Policy and Professional Practice
University of Keele
August 2010

Preface

Have you ever wondered what people talk about with their partners and families after a long day at work? Closer to home, what do you talk about when you drop the keys on the table and slump into a chair? Somewhere in those conversations, you will probably recognise the phrase: *'You won't believe what they did today!'*

The way people are managed at work not only affects their work performance; it leaks out into the rest of their lives. It affects their evenings, their weekends, their holidays and even their career choices. The reputation of managers in organisations, particularly in terms of how their decisions impact on their staff, will travel far and wide. Bear in mind that management is not a popularity contest and occasionally managers will be required to make decisions and bring about changes that people feel uneasy about. However, these decisions can *always* be made with integrity and respect. Many of the 'you won't believe what they did today' stories we hear about tend to focus on the sheer inexplicability of the management behaviour or its unfairness, insensitivity or complete detachment from the people most affected.

Now for the really scary question if you are a manager: what do you think your staff will be saying tonight when they get home and regale their family with the edited highlights of your management actions? You may have a good idea, or you may be blissfully ignorant, but whatever your answer, it should give you food for thought.

This book is for managers who want to get 'people management right'. It is written by two people who have had their share of good and indifferent people management, who have managed staff and who now make their living developing the people-management skills of others. We have gone home and muttered about our treatment and we have been the patient listeners whilst others have done their muttering. As a result of these experiences, one simple question emerges.

> What is it that we do to people at work that makes them so annoyed, so undervalued and so unwilling to give their best?

Both of us have had successful careers in healthcare management, leadership and management development and, latterly, as independent development consultants. We have both obtained master's degrees in management and change in complex organisations. These careers have brought us into regular contact with new managers, rising stars, world-weary managers, top executives and even those whose 'escape tunnel' has finally come up outside the perimeter fence and they have forged new careers.

We have also talked long into the night with the staff who work for and with these managers. Time after time we see that people management is absolutely vital to bottom-line performance and that routinely it is not done well. By this we do not mean that it is deliberately done badly, but that for many managers ignorance and the lack of meaningful feedback result in poor people management. The self-aware managers tell us that there are some skills they wish they had been given at the start. Their staff tell us that there are some skills that really would make the difference between them coming to work with a positive outlook and coming to work with a heavy heart. Unsurprisingly, the same topics come up again and again, and this book is designed to support the development of just those skills.

Andrew Scowcroft
Andrew Price
August 2010

About the authors

Andrew Price MSc, MHSM, DipHSM

Andrew's main focus is on leadership and team development, helping people to work positively and effectively with each other. He works in the public, private and voluntary sectors.

Andrew moved into consultancy after a career in NHS management. During this time he moved from hospital management into leadership development, and his final NHS role was as the acting chief executive of the Centre for Health Leadership.

Andrew has an MSc in Leadership and Organisation in the Public Sector from the University of the West of England. He also has a Diploma in Health Management and is a member of the Institute of Health Management. He has published in a number of journals including *Health Service Journal, Health Management* and *Public Policy Review*.

Andrew lives in Bristol and is married to Ruth, a Dance Movement Psychotherapist. They have two daughters. Andrew is currently Chair of One25, a Bristol based charity working with abused and disadvantaged women.

Andrew Scowcroft MA, MHSM, MCIPD, FInst LM

Andrew is an experienced and respected management development consultant and health service manager, with 37 years public sector experience, including 20 years as a self-financing consultant.

He is frequently engaged by the NHS and other public and private sector clients to provide a range of services, from training and development programmes through to executive coaching for top managers. Andrew has a strong commitment to releasing the potential of leaders and managers, and their organisations, and his development activities are extremely highly rated due to the practical nature of the material and its rapid transferability to the workplace.

With Andrew Price he has developed Vital Signs, a suite of foundational management skills programmes for managers, and has received endorsement from the Institute of Leadership and Management for these courses.

Andrew has a Diploma from the Institute of Health Services Management, BPS Level A and B certificates in Psychometric Testing, and an MA in Learning and Change in Organisations, University of West of England.

He is an Honorary Senior Tutor at Cardiff University, and a Visiting Fellow of the Welsh Institute for Health and Social Care, at the University of Glamorgan.

Andrew lives in Llantrisant, South Wales, is married to Ann, an Occupational Therapist, and they have two daughters.

Both Andrews can be contacted via www.developmentconsultancy.co.uk

Acknowledgements

In addition to our writing and consultancy work, we also run a short skills-based development programme called Vital Signs, which draws upon much of the material in this book. As a result of our experience delivering the Vital Signs programme, we have received valuable feedback on the importance of the topics we cover, how best to put across the key messages and how the advice given has transformed the lives of managers and their teams. We therefore wish to acknowledge our enormous debt to the more than 250 managers who have so far experienced Vital Signs and the client organisations that placed their faith in our abilities.

Our heartfelt thanks also go to a number of people whose encouragement and practical help has made this book possible. Nicola Hartnell in the Development Consultancy office has produced, and commented on, numerous drafts and always managed to keep us on track. Ashleigh Dunn, Kim Tovey and the late Professor Stephen Prosser were all immensely supportive in critiquing the work and making wise suggestions for change and enhancement.

Finally, thanks to our families – Ann, Claire and Hannah; Ruth, Abbie and Roanna. You have not only supported and shaped our lives and careers, but have also been extremely tolerant of the frequent drafting meetings, excessive coffee consumption and our unhealthy obsession with crouching over our laptops. Without you this book would simply not exist and for that support we are eternally grateful.

Dedicated to Stephen Prosser, friend, mentor and servant leader.

Introduction

Picture the scene

You are waiting to see your new family doctor. Someone in the waiting area whispers in your ear: 'You do know that they haven't had any training yet? Apparently they did well at interview and this is their first week in the job. I hear that if they struggle, or if enough people complain, they might be sent on a course.'

Most people would head for the door and find someone who did know what they were doing! It is simply incomprehensible, unacceptable and frankly dangerous for professionals to be let loose without some basic training followed by a demonstration of their minimum standard of competence. Why then is the management of people all too often seen as different? Do we think so little of the new manager, and the staff whose lives and work they are about to influence, that their training can wait, sometimes until years after their appointment, sometimes forever? Perhaps we do not see management as either important enough or even a profession. Our approach to preparing new managers certainly gives the clear impression that the work is unimportant and straightforward, with an expectation that the necessary skills can be picked up 'on the job'.

We think new managers, *and* those they manage, deserve better. Therefore, this book is aimed directly at the person who, for whatever reason, finds themselves managing, or about to manage, others. This might be due to a wished-for promotion, or it may simply be that looking after some staff comes with starting a new project. It may even be that an internal reorganisation has 'bolted-on' people management to an existing technical role.

This book does not set out to cover every management facet. There are several excellent and thoughtful manuals that address the increasingly complex world of management and leadership. Neither does it take just one topic and provide intensive theoretical or step-by-step advice on mastering that single subject. Again, there are many first-class single-issue books available.

In this book, we identify the critical few skills that a manager will need *from day one*, skills that will allow them to settle into the role, gain self-confidence *and* the respect of their staff, survive and thrive in those early weeks, and so create a steady platform for acquiring and mastering new skills in the future.

What it tries to do is to set the manager on a well-managed and supported path of continuing professional development by providing practical approaches to the common challenges they will face as they get to grips with the job, the people and the culture. Once they have developed that confidence and once they have some progress on which to build, they can then engage with some of the more complex, strategic, financial and political issues waiting for them around the corner.

The areas covered in the book will provide you with answers to some important questions, and some practical ways of demonstrating your skills.

Part 1 looks at the way managers engage with their staff. It contains four chapters that look at managing the whole team, looking after individuals and managing the change process.

Part 2 offers advice on some technical management disciplines; specifically, managing meetings, making presentations and writing management reports.

The key questions for each topic are given below.

PART 1: DEALING WITH PEOPLE

Chapter 1: Dealing with people

How do you take on and begin to harness the skills and potential of your new team? How indeed do you cope with being promoted from within your peers and suddenly having to 'be the boss'? How do you find out where the team is strong and where it needs development?

Chapter 2: Dealing with individuals

Whatever your organisation's manual tells you about the process and documentation of appraisal, how do you prepare for and run that first performance review session? What do you say, who takes the lead, and why should people participate anyway? Why do some sessions start out okay but fall apart later on? Why is tackling a performance issue so sensitive, and what do you say and do to keep the process dignified, respectful and productive?

Chapters 3 and 4: Leading change/Tools for change

What do you do when there is a need for change, or an opportunity to do things differently in your team or section, but previous change strategies have produced anxiety, animosity or even rebellion? Why do some people go for new things and others look the other way? How can you make effective change stick?

PART 2: MANAGEMENT DISCIPLINES
Chapter 5: So many meetings!

Why are so many meetings perceived by participants and onlookers alike as a waste of time, and what can you do to lead a successful one from the start?

Chapter 6: Making confident presentations

How can you put your case across to staff, meetings, board members and external agencies without losing your nerve and your notes, and without hiding behind flashy slides?

Chapter 7: Effective management reports

What do you put in a short management report that will get results without curing the reader's insomnia?

Chapter 8: Over to you

This final chapter identifies some learning and review techniques that readers can use to sharpen their thinking, and concludes with an invitation to transform your people management practice, for the benefit of you, your team and the organisation in which you work.

Time after time managers and staff tell us that good management is evidenced by effective people-management, confident communication and well-managed change. In contrast, poor management (as reported through things like staff satisfaction surveys, confidential interviews and 360° feedback) is usually accompanied by anecdotes about insensitive people management, timid or arrogant new managers, worthless or misguided communication and clumsy change management. In the face of such consistent messages, we believe that this book can make a major contribution to improving both the practice and the reputation of local management in the workplace.

The book can be used as a stand-alone guide and reference, and we hope that organisations and employers will see fit to attach it to every first-level management job offer letter. It may be too much to ask that it could be given to those with management potential to help them decide whether to take the plunge, but we live in hope. The book is also being used as a companion to the aforementioned five-day Vital Signs programme, run by the authors.

But what if you are not a 'new manager'? Our work also reveals that many of the more experienced managers in organisations slipped through the management training net in earlier years and are now in the sorts of positions where 'going on a management course' may be socially awkward or somewhat career limiting. Nevertheless, they recognise that they don't always handle issues well and would benefit from advice and guidance. Typically these are high-status technical professionals who have embraced management following promotion or as part of broadening their organisational experience. Regardless of their route into management they still feel under prepared.

We therefore hope that these more experienced managers would not be averse to dipping in and out of this book as a way of quality checking their current practice and picking up some new approaches.

At all times when reading this book and when going about your daily management tasks, please remember that you, and the people you manage, are human beings. They have complex needs, they do not act like robots, nor should they. Just because you are their manager this does not guarantee that every technique will work first time, every time. Don't assume that every employee can be completely 'worked out' and then become putty in your hands.

True learning about management does not come from consistently chalking up successful tactics and plans. True learning comes from grappling with an issue, reflecting on what didn't work as well as what did, and honing your craft as a result of your experiences. As Huxley once wrote: '*Experience is not what happens to you, but what you do with what happens to you*' (Aldous Huxley. *Texts and Pretexts*. London: Chatto and Windus; 1932).

So, whether you are thinking about going for a management post, have just been appointed to your first position, looked up one day and realised that there are people around you that might just be relying on you for management support, or you simply want reassurance that what you thought *was* the right approach *is* the right approach, we know you will find this book helpful.

Now read on – your staff will thank you for it.

PART 1

Dealing with people

CHAPTER 1

Dealing with people

TEAMS: THEY ARE CENTRAL TO OUR EXPERIENCE OF WORK BUT SO LITTLE UNDERSTOOD

The existence of any organisation of a size greater than one person is proof of our persistent belief that we can achieve more by working together than we can on our own. Michael West from Aston University points out that it is our ability to work cooperatively that has enabled humans to make such remarkable progress, and that our extraordinary achievements in science or exploration have been largely made by teams.[1] Teams have conquered Everest, mapped the human genome and produced the Authorised version of the Bible. Teams have put men on the moon and split the atom. But despite all the evidence of the creative potential of teams, we keep finding organisations who begrudge the time and effort needed to develop them. In this chapter we'll underline the importance of teams, set out the foundations of effective teamwork and look at the different ways people contribute to team success. At the end of the chapter we'll give you a simple framework to use in reviewing your team.

HOW DO TEAMS AFFECT US?

We've often asked people about their experiences in teams.

'Think of the worst teams you've been in,' we say, 'and tell us what characterised them and what impact they had on you.' Regardless of their profession or organisation, people tend to say the same things. The worst teams they've been in were characterised by:

➤ poor communication
➤ unclear roles
➤ unhappiness and even bullying
➤ members 'watching their back'

➤ cliques and politics
➤ poor leadership – either oppressive or non-existent.

People in these teams:
➤ dreaded going into work
➤ experienced fear, sickness and stress
➤ wanted to leave the organisation
➤ did just enough to get by.

THE LEGACY OF TEAMS

When we ask people about their experiences in teams we are often taken aback by the stories we are told of victimisation, humiliation and conflict, often involving senior professional staff, and by how long the memories of such experiences persist. Although many years may have passed, anger or resentment about being part of a dysfunctional team is not far below the surface and, therefore, liable to still influence the way such people currently behave in teams. We have also often noticed a change in the mood of these groups when they think about their best teams. Body language and the tone of the discussion reflect pleasure or excitement. The legacy of teams is, for good or ill, very long-lived.

We then ask people to think of the characteristics of the best teams they have been in, and what impact these teams had on them and their work. Again, people tend to say the same sorts of things. Good teams:
➤ work towards a common purpose
➤ give every member a part to play
➤ work flexibly
➤ have a sense of identity.

The impact of these teams on their members was, not surprisingly, very positive. They tended to experience:
➤ enjoyment
➤ a sense of achievement
➤ high levels of commitment
➤ support from other team members
➤ less stress and sick leave.

The comments made by the groups we have worked with are echoed in research into teams. It seems we have the very best and very worst of our work experience in team settings.

THE INVISIBLE LEADER

We've noticed that people seem to mention leadership more often when they are talking about bad teams than when they are talking about good teams. When describing poor teams they often identify defective leadership as a cause, but when they describe their best teams they tend to talk about things that are the results of good leadership – purpose, role clarity, flexibility – rather than about leadership itself. It reminds us of the saying attributed to Lao Tzu (600–531BC): *'A leader is best when people barely know he exists, when his work is done, his aim fulfilled, they will say: we did it ourselves.'*

GOOD TEAMS: JUST A BONUS?

But does any of this really matter? If people feel fear, stress and confusion, or alternatively a sense of purpose and commitment, does this significantly affect their work? If the answer is no, hard-pressed bosses might be forgiven for neglecting the development of their teams. But if the answer is yes, we should make a conscious effort to create and maintain good teams.

So let's consider the evidence. First subjectively. Imagine you visit two hospital departments as a patient. In one the staff seem happy, purposeful and flexible. In the other they seem stressed and defensive. Assuming that each department is staffed by fully qualified professionals, in which department would you expect to receive the better care?

Second, an example from recent history. In 1998 the Government set up an inquiry into children's heart surgery at the Bristol Royal Infirmary. Public concern about the deaths of children followed by disciplinary action against several medical staff indicated that something had gone wrong. The inquiry was chaired by Professor Ian Kennedy and considered evidence from nearly 600 witnesses. The report of the inquiry included the following observation:

> There was poor teamwork and this had implications for performance and outcome. The crucial importance of effective teamwork in this complex area of surgery was very widely recognized. Effective teamwork did not always exist at the BRI. There were logistical reasons for this: for example the cardiologists could not be everywhere. The point is that everyone just carried on.[2]

So, while other factors were involved, poor teamwork had influenced the standard of care given to children. What is more, despite widespread recognition of the importance of teamwork 'everyone just carried on'. The cost of this unwillingness to tackle poor teamwork was high.

Again, in 2010, another inquiry into the deaths of babies following heart surgery, this time at the Oxford Radcliffe NHS Trust, found that the lack of teamwork between the surgeons adversely affected the work of the unit.[6]

Finally, research with 400 teams and 7000 staff in the NHS showed that the benefits of effective teams include higher-quality care, more innovations and lower levels of stress among team members. The research also highlighted a significant statistical relationship between the percentage of hospital staff working in effective teams and patient mortality.[3]

So it seems that not only are effective teams healthier, more enjoyable contexts to work in, they are also more productive and innovative, contributing to higher quality services.

TEAMS AND GROUPS

There is a tendency in organisations to call any grouping of staff a team. This can lead to confusion and even conflict as the 'team' searches for a purpose and function to justify its existence. We find it is helpful to distinguish between groups and teams. The main difference is that members of *teams* have to work together closely and supportively to achieve a shared goal. For some purposes, a group is the best solution. For many years a number of training managers from separate health organisations used to meet together. Functioning as a *group* – exchanging information and enabling smaller interest groups to form – the gatherings worked well. But when some members tried to make the group behave like a team and establish a unique shared purpose and collaborative working, it became apparent that something artificial was being created. Most group members, whose first loyalty was to their organisation, resisted being tied into a team. Moreover there was no clear team task. The result was misunderstanding and ill feeling.

BUILDING A GOOD TEAM: YOUR MOST IMPORTANT TASK

There is plenty of evidence that the quality of teamwork is a major influence on the service an organisation provides. On top of this, being in a good team makes us less stressed, more innovative and more committed. For all these reasons we believe that developing an effective team is perhaps the most important task of any manager. But if this is true, why are there so many ineffective teams and why, like at the Bristol Royal Infirmary, when teamwork is poor, do we just carry on? It is as if we see being in a well-managed team as a bonus or an act of God, whereas we should see it as a basic right of every employee.

REASONS FOR INEFFECTIVE TEAMS

1 **Great teams don't happen by accident.**

Effective teams don't just happen, they have to be shaped and developed. Even where you have a group of committed, flexible and competent people, you will still have to put thought and effort into developing a team.

2   **Building teams is simple . . . but not easy.**
The elements of successful team leadership are not complicated or extremely intellectually challenging. You do not need to be a genius to master what causes teams to flourish and what makes them flounder. But you do need character. You will need to persevere in the face of misunderstanding or opposition. No wonder many managers prefer to focus on the technical parts of their job because they are less demanding. We suspect that when managers claim to be too busy to develop their team, it is often a justification for avoiding issues that demand character as well as skill.

3   **Delayed impact.**
It seems that the closer an action is to its consequences, the easier it is to learn from that action. Touching something hot is immediately painful so we learn not to do it. The impact of either developing or ignoring your team is less immediate. There is no instant and obvious 'bottom-line' result of carrying out a good appraisal, clarifying team roles or agreeing objectives, so it is tempting to neglect team development for more pressing but in the end less-important tasks.

THE FOUNDATIONS OF EFFECTIVE TEAMWORK

Regardless of what sector you work in or what type of staff make up the team, we suggest that there are five foundations for effective working that all teams need.

1   **Purpose: clear, shared and worthwhile.**
Teams must have a common purpose. This should explain the reason for the existence of the team and it should be something worth working towards. However, we have learned never to assume that teams are clear about their purpose. In one team we worked with, our question about purpose was greeted with amusement if not derision: *'We're the top management team. Its obvious what we do!'* As we interviewed the members though, we found a variety of ideas about team purpose. For some the team's role was to focus on the big picture and give overall vision and direction for the organisation. Others insisted that their role was to be the operational decision-making hub of the company. Both were valid purposes, but as we watched the team we could see how differing ideas about their purpose pulled the agenda in different directions, leaving all the members frustrated.

Teams often confuse their purpose with their day-to-day activity but there is an important difference; activity is what you do, *purpose* is why you do it. Having a clear shared purpose enables each team member to see their role in the context of something greater than themselves. For example, take two clerical staff working in a hospital. One has simply been asked to collect certain pieces of information from medical records and send them to someone else. The other has exactly the same task, but understands their role to be part of a team who are studying different ways of treating a particular illness so that patients can be treated more safely and more effectively. While the task is identical, one sees the greater purpose and understands why it is important to have accurate and timely information. For the other it is simply a chore, with no sense of rhyme or reason. Which one is likely to do a better job?

We suggest two ways of getting to the real purpose of your team. First, think about what you do and then ask yourself why you do it. If your team runs a clinic, why does that clinic exist? Your first answer might be 'to treat patients'. If so, keep asking why. What does that treatment enable? A team who provided mobility aids to patients realised that their purpose was not to provide wheelchairs or electric scooters but to enable their patients to live full and unrestricted lives. This is a good example of purpose because it is clear, motivational and, importantly, hard to achieve. The other way to get to your purpose is to ask yourself what bad things would happen if your team and the service it provides did not exist. What impact on people would this have?

Distinguishing purpose from activity is so important. Not only does it motivate the team and guide decisions but, it also helps it to innovate and change, to seize new opportunities. The mobility-aids team we mentioned above are more likely to be open to new ways of removing physical restrictions for their patients as new technologies emerge. They realise that providing wheelchairs, etc. is not their purpose, just the current best way of achieving it. If better ways come along, old ways can be discarded or adapted. One of the reasons some teams and organisations find change hard is that they can see no further than what they currently do.

2 **Clear roles**

In our school-yard football matches there were no team positions. A thundering herd of boys would simply follow the ball around the playground, everyone trying to be the goal-scoring hero. Some management teams and team meetings are little better, with everyone competing for airtime and no attempt to distinguish roles or play to individual strengths. In the boardroom as well as the playground, this lack of clarity leads to confusion, wasted resources and even the occasional scuffle! Like the team who fly a plane (pilot, navigator, co-pilot.) or the team around an operating table (surgeon, nurse, anaesthetist), teams work best when each person knows how they fit in to the overall team task. Before you start using any fancy management techniques, we guarantee you can make a difference to your team by making sure everyone knows what they are supposed to be doing and why. We also guarantee that your team is not as clear about this as you think they are!

3 **Feedback on individual performance.**
We cover appraisal elsewhere in this book, but for now let's just acknowledge a paradox of management – we all want to know how we are doing, but we feel uncomfortable when we have to tell others. To cover our discomfort, we avoid doing appraisal or we formalise it into a paper/computer exercise. This is unfortunate, because well-handled appraisal is one of the most powerful and positive tools available to the manager.

4 **Feedback on team performance.**
This has two levels. First, the team needs to have clear goals, so that the achievement of these goals can be used to measure progress and success. Second, teams need to reflect on their performance *as a team* and assess how effectively they work together and the quality of their communication. We would suggest that every 6–9 months you give your team an opportunity to reflect and to plan ahead (*see* 'Vision of the future' in Chapter 4). A skilled facilitator is useful to make sure the process is positive and helpful. The sorts of questions the team would address are:
— 'Over the last 6 months, what has worked well and what has worked badly?'
— 'Is our purpose still relevant, clear and shared?'
— 'Where do we need to be in 12 months time?'
— 'What do we need to do now to make sure we get there?'
The focus needs to be on learning, not blaming, and the team leader needs to set the tone by being honest, by showing respect to team members and by avoiding cynicism.

5 **Clear leadership.**
Becoming a good leader does not happen automatically when we take up a leadership position, any more than becoming a good parent happens as soon as we have children. Both roles take time and practice and both are often done badly. There needs to be clarity about how the team is led, even if different people take the lead on different issues.

THE CHALLENGE OF BEING PROMOTED FROM WITHIN THE TEAM

Going from colleague to boss can be a difficult transition and many participants on our Vital Signs course admit to having found it traumatic. But there are ways you can ease the transition.

Make it discussable

You will encounter a subtle but profound shift in the nature of your relationships within the team. Saying something like 'this feels a bit weird to me, what about you?' can allow others to articulate the awkwardness of the situation and, by talking about it, make it less awkward.

Don't play favourites

You may need to have a private chat to your friends in the team and explain that, while the friendship is unaffected, you cannot be seen to favour one team member more than another. This may mean that your routine of always having a catch up over morning coffee may need to finish or be done in a way that is more inclusive.

Messiah complex

Think twice before you organise a big, special meeting to announce your promotion and outline your world-changing vision, you may just end up looking silly.

Keep the team informed of your movements

Often promotion will mean that you spend more time away from the team. Unless you explain why you are absent, some will unfairly assume that you are absent from where the real work is getting done. Let the team know that you are continuing to fight the good fight but that you need to do it in meetings, conferences or other events that are away from the workplace.

THE IMPORTANCE OF DIFFERENCE

Team skills

In teams, much of the value lies in the differences between people. This is easy to appreciate as we think of the skills we bring. For example, orchestras and expedition teams rely on having people who can bring different skills. No one would criticise the cook on a polar expedition for not knowing enough about satellite communications, and no orchestra would sack a violinist for not knowing how to play percussion. In fact the excellence of such teams depends on each person being given the room to make their unique contribution. In the same way, organisational teams benefit from having a range of skills appropriate to the task of the team.

A typical senior management team might bring together people with skills in accountancy, personnel management, production and planning. A team planning a new building may have an architect, an engineer, a builder and a project manager. The effectiveness of the team depends on each member being able and willing to make their contribution. Each person brings a different perspective and insight into the issues faced by the team. From time to time there may be tension when these different perspectives suggest different courses of action, but as long as the team has a clear sense of purpose and good leadership, these tensions, far from being destructive, help the team work more creatively. The wise team welcomes the different approaches each person brings, knowing that its decisions will benefit. It would clearly be foolish to try and promote the smooth running of the team by choosing people who all have the same skill! The likely result would be an unbalanced team.

Team roles and the myth of the 'team player'

While most people can see the value of having different skills or professions on a team, there is less understanding of the need to have people who bring different personalities and behaviour. This is exemplified in the way the phrase 'team player' is so often quoted in job adverts and job specifications as if it were a single personality type. In the same way that we welcome a variety of skills and professional backgrounds, we should also welcome a variety of personalities and ways of seeing the world.

Hollywood understands this point better than the average boardroom. In every film about teams, whether it is *Ocean's Eleven*, *Kelly's Heroes* or *The Lord of the Rings*, we see how the interplay of different personalities is crucial to the team's success or failure. In *The Lord of the Rings*, Gandalf's wisdom and vision is not enough. He needs Frodo's idealism and courage and Sam's single-minded stubbornness to complete the task. In *Ocean's Eleven*, success hinges on Danny Ocean's ability to hold together a team who, as well as having different skills, are very different people. Some are strategic, others are obsessed with detail. Some are careful and considered, others more impetuous. Their differences are not only a source of tension, they are essential to the mission. What such films illustrate is that there is no single type of person who is a 'team player'. Rather, it is the differences between us that make teams effective.

Thankfully, we don't have to rely on Hollywood for proof of the importance of diversity of personality and thinking styles in teams. A research-based model has been provided by Raymond Meredith Belbin, whose concept of team roles has become an essential part of so many training courses and books about management. Belbin coined the term 'team role' to refer to a person's 'tendency to behave, contribute and interrelate with others at work in certain and distinctive ways'.[4] It is important to distinguish between a person's *team* role, which is about behaviour, and their *functional* role, which is about professional or technical skills and knowledge. Hence two people with the same functional role, doctor perhaps, may have very different ways of behaving and interacting with people at work. Same functional role, different team roles.

TEAM PLAYERS: THE SEARCH FOR THE HOLY GRAIL

Some time ago, both of us were involved in selecting graduates for fast-track management programmes. We would design assessment centres, often lasting two or three days, and observe the candidates in a variety of situations to see how closely they matched a set of predetermined competences. Some of these competences were related to team behaviour. On reflection, we were looking for people who possessed an impossible combination of personality features: dynamic, decisive, influential, innovative, sociable strategists who were also sensitive and reflective listeners with a grasp of detail. Indisputably all these characteristics are desirable, but we rarely find them in the same person – and certainly not at the same time!

Belbin's careful study of over 200 teams at Henley Management College led him to the conclusion that the balance of team roles is crucial to the success of a team.[5] Having people with the right technical skills is not enough. He identified nine clusters of behaviors, which he called team roles, and suggested that a balance of all nine roles is needed for a team to be effective. This doesn't mean that each team needs at least nine people! Most of us will be capable of discharging several of these roles, but the mix of preferred roles will differ from person to person.

One of Belbin's most valuable insights is that each team role has a number of important strengths and some weaknesses. He calls these 'allowable weaknesses'. This is a useful reminder that all of us have areas of both strength and weakness and that no one, no matter how senior or successful, can be the mythical 'team player' – excellent in every role.

TABLE 1.1 Belbin's team roles

Role	Contribution	Allowable weaknesses
Plant	Creative, imaginative, unorthodox. Solves difficult problems.	Ignores details. Too preoccupied to communicate effectively.
Resource investigator	Extrovert, enthusiastic, communicative. Explores opportunities. Develops contacts.	Over-optimistic. Loses interest once initial enthusiasm has passed.
Coordinator	Mature, confident, a good chairperson. Clarifies goals, promotes decision-making, delegates well.	Can be seen as manipulative. Delegates personal work.
Shaper	Challenging, dynamic, thrives on pressure. Has the drive and courage to overcome obstacles.	Can provoke others. Hurts people's feelings.
Monitor evaluator	Sober, strategic and discerning. Sees all options. Judges accurately.	Lacks drive and ability to inspire others. Overly critical.
Teamworker	Cooperative, mild, perceptive and diplomatic. Listens, builds, averts friction, calms the waters.	Indecisive in crunch situations. Can be easily influenced.

(continued)

Role	Contribution	Allowable weaknesses
Implementer	Disciplined, reliable, conservative and efficient. Turns ideas into practical actions.	Somewhat inflexible. Slow to respond to new possibilities.
Completer	Painstaking, conscientious, anxious. Searches out errors and omissions. Delivers on time.	Inclined to worry unduly. Reluctant to delegate. Can be a nit-picker.
Specialist	Single-minded, self-starting, dedicated. Provides knowledge and skills in rare supply.	Contributes only on a narrow front. Dwells on technicalities. Overlooks the big picture.

Source: adapted from Raymond Meredith Belbin, *Team Roles at Work*.

Working with team roles

We have found that Belbin's concept of team roles is a really useful tool in understanding what is going on in a team. It underlines the importance of valuing people who think and behave in different ways to ourselves. We may find this annoying from time to time but Belbin's work reminds us that this difference is part of the strength of the team. Here are three questions to ask yourself

1 **What are my preferred roles?**

   Through reflection and talking with colleagues, consider which team roles best reflect the way you behave in teams. If you have access to the Belbin questionnaire this would also be useful. Be realistic – you won't be strong in all nine roles! On the other hand, everyone has strengths, and someone will have preferences that complement and balance yours.

2 **What are my least preferred roles?**

   This will direct you to areas that might be blind spots, or it might illustrate the types of behaviours that frustrate you when you encounter them in others.

3 **What roles are present in your team?**

   Think about your team. What team roles are most obvious in the way it works? What about the roles that are less obvious? Is each person encouraged to make their team roles contribution or are the less common roles squeezed out?

FROM SCEPTIC TO CYNIC: AN EXAMPLE OF FRUSTRATED TEAM ROLES

A former colleague of ours had many years' experience coupled with an analytical mind and a knack of bursting people's bubbles when they strayed too far from the path of logic. Perhaps because of this tendency to expose flaws in his colleagues' thinking, he attracted an unfavourable reputation as a negative thinker. Increasingly, he was sidelined and ignored, remaining a middle manager as his contemporaries were promoted to senior posts. As a result, his scepticism, which potentially was of great value to the organisation in testing out ideas, turned into cynicism and he eventually left the organisation to take early retirement after becoming 'displaced' in a restructuring. The organisation had lost a much-needed 'monitor evaluator' because it failed to recognise and reward his contribution. Sceptics are not always easy to work with but they can bring a healthy dose of realism to a team that might otherwise begin to believe its own publicity.

THE FOUR Ps: DIAGNOSING TEAM ISSUES

It's easy to see when a team isn't working well, but much harder to put your finger on why. Like a good doctor we have to be able to separate symptoms from causes. In Chapter 4 we'll talk about how something called 'systems thinking' helps us do this, but for now let's just agree that merely attacking the symptoms of team problems is about as useful as just putting a plaster over a wound that needs stitches.

Staying with the medical metaphor for a moment, the problem with just responding to the obvious and immediate issues is that the place where we experience pain is not always the place where the real problem is. Pain in your arm might indicate heart problems, and pain in the shoulder can be the result of an inflamed gall bladder. In the same way, an apparent personality clash in a team may be the result of two members having unclear or incompatible roles. Appealing for calm or threatening disciplinary action may suppress the symptoms but the problem will remain. Poor attendance at team gatherings may be nothing to do with diary management or the time of the meeting. It may well indicate that some members find meetings to be uncomfortable or of little value, in which case a three-line whip may only increase frustration.

The four Ps are simple enough to be memorable but have enough detail to guide you through a robust analysis of the state of your team. We recommend that you use them as a checklist, working through each of the sections in turn and answering the questions with your team in mind.

TABLE 1.2 The four Ps

Area	Useful questions
Purpose – what the team is for	• Is the team's purpose clear and shared? • Is a team the right answer for this task? • Is the team's purpose seen as useful and therefore motivational?
People – how members contribute	• Does the team have the skills and knowledge it needs? • Do all members have clear and compatible roles? • Are all of Belbin's team roles covered?

(continued)

Area	Useful questions
Procedures – formal systems underpinning the team	• Are there effective systems in place to support communication between members? • Meetings? • Individual appraisal? • Allocation of work?
Processes – how the team works together	• Leadership – how is the team led? Is this clear and agreed? • Learning – how does the team review and improve its performance? • Strategy and planning – how does the team shape its future?

CONCLUSION

We hope that we've communicated the importance of good teams. We'd go so far as to say that for most managers, leading their team to a place where it works effectively is the most important part of their role. If we can do this, motivation, creativity, productivity and quality are likely to follow. But before we leave this subject, a word of caution. Using the models and checklists we have offered in this chapter, you will almost certainly have identified areas that require change. Don't assume that your colleagues see things the same way. You run the risk of trying to implement the right changes in the wrong way. Chapter 4 will give you practical guidance on how to introduce and manage change.

REFERENCES

1 West M. *Effective Teamwork*. 2nd ed. Malden: Blackwell; 2004.

2 Bristol Royal Infirmary Inquiry. *Learning from Bristol: the report of the public inquiry into children's heart surgery at the Bristol Royal Infirmary 1984–1995*. Command Paper CM 5207. London: The Stationery Office; 2001.

3 Borrill C, West M, Dawson J, *et al. Team Working and Effectiveness in Health Care: findings from the Health Care Team Effectiveness Project*. Birmingham: Aston Centre for Health Service Organisation Research, Aston University (Psychological Therapies Research Centre, University of Leeds) Humans Communications Research Centre, University of Glasgow; 2002.

4 Belbin RM. *Team Roles at Work*. Oxford: Butterworth-Heinemann; 1993.

5 You can read about this in *Management Teams: why they succeed or fail* by RM Belbin (Oxford: Butterworth-Heinemann; 1996). Also, www.belbin.com links you to other team roles resources.

6 NHS South Central. *Review of Paediatric Cardiac Services at the Oxford Radcliffe Hospitals NHS Trust*. London: NHS South Central; 2010. See www.southcentral.nhs.uk/document_store/128040127741_orh_paediatric_review.pdf.

CHAPTER 2

Dealing with individuals

LEADING INDIVIDUALS

So far we have looked at some of the characteristics of your team and how you can help team members work effectively together. We now turn our attention to the responsibilities you have to each individual in that team, and how you can get the best out of each one. Anecdotal evidence suggests that it is the relationship a person has with their manager, more so than with their fellow team members, that will determine whether they stay or leave. That relationship will also heavily influence how hard and effectively a person works if they do stay.

This chapter looks at five main areas of the manager–employee relationship.

1 First we will explore some elements of *motivation*, because managers need to know how to create the right environment for each person to give of their best.
2 Second is the issue of *appraisal*. Different organisations and employers have different names for this process and, to some, the word appraisal is a little outdated. Whatever it is called, spending protected time with staff discussing their performance, personal development, ideas for the future and giving constructive feedback, is central to the manager's role and we discuss some of main ingredients in this chapter.
3 The third area is that of *personal development planning*. Many sophisticated tools exist to support this process, but we believe in keeping things simple. Furthermore, given that the whole person comes to work, it is the whole person that should be given the opportunity to develop.
4 Fourth is the thorny issue of tackling *poor or sub-optimal performance*. Our experience is that addressing poor performance is either avoided for as long as possible or is too hastily escalated to bring in formal disciplinary or capability procedures. This chapter will show you how to intervene quickly, sensitively and constructively, with the sole intention of returning the employee to form as soon as possible.

5   The fifth and final element in the relationship between manager and staff is *the human relationship itself*. In part this involves the manager adapting their 'management style' to take account of the needs of the individual at any point of time. Traditional management thinking has encouraged managers to adopt one particular style – democratic, participative, benevolent, autocratic, etc. We think this is unhelpful and fails to take into account the whole person, the changing nature of their lives and careers, and any alterations in their motivational drivers. Improving the relationship also requires the manager to spot those occasions where they find themselves in self-perpetuating loops of behaviour with particular members of staff, loops that produce unhelpful outcomes and entrenched positions being taken by both parties. We will show how these episodes start and what the manager can do to prevent them, or get out of them once started.

As you read this chapter you may find yourself thinking, 'All of this requires time – where am I going to find the time needed to do all these things?'

Our answer is somewhat blunt but etched with personal experience.

Finding the time for your staff is the essence of your job! Managers are really good at finding the time to fire-fight, to solve the crises as they arise and to rescue their teams from the abyss time and time again. Strange then that they cannot find the time to put the foundations in place at the start, and then keep in touch with staff to spot the early signs of trouble. We would go further and say that the *first* responsibility of a manager is the people they manage. To them, you represent the whole management system of your organisation; therefore the interest you show in them demonstrates that organisation's view of their staff. If we had a pound for every time we have heard the words 'our people are our most valuable asset', we would both be retired by now. Sadly, the day-to-day behaviour of many organisations gives those words a hollow ring, and your approach to the individuals you manage will be used by staff as a litmus test of their employer's view of them.

Now let's look at each of these five areas in more detail.

Motivation

Theories abound on the subject of motivation, but you did not pick up this book to learn about theories. So let us get right to the heart of the subject.

Consider this question. *What factors are affecting your engagement with this task (reading the book) right now?*

If it helps, make some notes in the box on the next page. Don't overthink or self-edit at this stage, simply jot down all the factors (positive and negative) that are impacting on the act of reading this section.

You'll probably find that a variety of things are helping or hindering you as you read. Some might be to do with the book itself (style of writing, relevance), some might be purely physical (light levels, comfort) and some are unconnected issues that are competing for your attention (work deadlines, crying children). History might be playing a part – the last management book you read was helpful/boring/confusing, etc.

When we ask participants on our programmes to answer this same question about the session they are taking part in, typical responses include:

Work pressures, wondering what to eat tonight, hoping to learn something useful, hot, cold, unwell, hung-over, wanting to participate, still thinking about yesterday's meeting, planning for difficult chat with the boss tomorrow, childminder was late, kids not well . . .

One of the things that this exercise reinforces is that we are human, that our lives are complex, and that however professional we are it is difficult to simply switch off one part of our lives when we engage with another part. The point here is that the staff we manage are exactly the same – they have complex lives and their level of motivation (or engagement with their work) will be affected by many factors. Your simple acceptance of this fact will immediately make you a more reasonable and sensitive manager.

You may not be able to influence any of those personal external factors, but you can at least appreciate that a member of your staff can be up one day and down the next, fully engaged one minute and a little preoccupied the next. This is not an excuse to condone unacceptable performance or bad behaviour – these do need to be tackled (*see* 'Tackling poor performance', p. 31) – but acknowledging the fact that we are human can go a long way towards making staff feel valued and appreciated.

If we look now at some of the more explicit motivators, the first thing to say is that what gets your staff to come to work is not necessarily the thing that will make them work well once they get there.

Second, every single person you employ or manage will have different motivations from one day to the next, and some will find their motivators changing throughout their career. Therefore the astute manager is aware of both the general motivators at work and the make up of each person they manage.

A pragmatic summary of much of the research on motivation is that there are three main drivers – economic, intrinsic and social.

The bad news is that for many junior and middle managers they have little or no control over the first of these! The good news is that it is the other two that tend to be more effective in improving long-term performance.

Economic motivators, as the name suggests, include the pursuit of money and material gain, either as a statement of social position and wealth, or as a way of securing other goals and objectives outside of the workplace. We know that our pay, when compared to the demands of our jobs (or even when compared to others around us), may make us dissatisfied with those jobs and may make us seek alternative employment. However, it seems that money is not very effective as a long-term motivator and, interestingly, has never appeared in the responses to the question we asked at the start of this section. Imagine you felt that your value to your employer was not being reflected in your current pay. Now assume that your employer agreed, and, using the appropriate mechanism, your pay was increased by £2 000pa. The money has perhaps persuaded you to stay, but will it make you work any harder? Probably not, after the first few days of feeling positive towards your employer. However, your good fortune may have a negative impact on your colleagues, who now feel undervalued themselves.

> We accept that some bonus schemes, or piece-rate payment systems, do show a clear relationship between effort and financial reward, but the principle remains that for most waged or salaried employees, money is not directly related to performance. Indeed at the time of writing (2010), the worldwide banking industry is under severe scrutiny because its bonus culture seems to be unrelated to overall performance and, arguably, has even contributed to irresponsible risk taking.

For most people, money (as a motivator) gets you to the 'factory gate' or helps you decide to go to a different factory gate, but it does not make you work more effectively once you pass through those gates. For that, we have to look at the other two motivators.

Intrinsic motivation comes from the sense of worth and value attached to the job itself, its purpose and meaning, its impact on those affected, and from the intellectual and/or physical challenges it contains. A craftsperson who takes satisfaction from a job well done is experiencing intrinsic motivation. For some, it is the fact that considerable training and experience is required that gives the job some of its intrinsic value (even if some people do not see the job itself as important to society). For others it is a sense of vocation (paid or unpaid) that just makes the job 'a good thing to do'.

Managers have considerable influence over the nature of employees' jobs and so can impact significantly on the intrinsic nature of their work. Whilst not excusing avoidable poor working conditions and uncompetitive pay, the intrinsic motivation of some jobs is enough to have the person accepting considerable hardships. The difficult environments faced by many overseas aid and development agencies, coupled with the generally low levels of pay and working conditions, are self-evident. Yet many people choose to undertake this work for part or all of their careers, and the intrinsic motivation more than compensates for the low financial rewards.

Social motivation is the sense of community and belonging that comes from a workplace that not only encourages workers to come to work but to go the extra mile once there.

We know of one lottery winner who, although scooping £1.1m whilst off sick, could not wait to return to work at her local hospital laundry (earning £6 per hour). She explained that it was a big part of her life, and her boss described her as a valued and respected member of the team. Whilst it could be argued that there is some intrinsic motivation in the work (turning dirty sheets into clean sheets for ill people), it was surely the social motivation that was drawing her back to work as her friends all worked there – she certainly did not need the money. One year after her win, she was still there!

The social aspect of motivation has arguably been assuming greater significance as the nature of society in Western Europe has been changing over the last two generations. If we go back to the age of our grandparents, even the extended family members would have lived close to each other, in the same or adjacent streets. They would have gained much of their sense of community and social cohesion from the world outside their work. Their economic motivators were met by their workplace and, whilst some jobs were very short on intrinsic value, the promise of community after work kept them going. For the current generation, we are likely to live some distance from even immediate family members. Beyond the family unit, as membership of community organisations, clubs, societies, churches, etc. continue to fall, we may look for and find that sense of community in our workplace and with our work colleagues.

> **MOTIVATED BY MEANING**
>
> Margaret Wheatley and Myron Kellner-Rogers[1] remind us that 'we are always seeking meaning in what we do. We find this in small tasks, in large causes and in relationships' (p. 92). Maybe in a society where the political, religious and cultural ideas that used to explain and give meaning to our lives are increasingly questioned or discarded, many look to their work to give their lives a sense of meaning or purpose. Wise managers who help their teams connect to a sense of meaning in their work will be rewarded (and challenged!) by levels of creativity and commitment that go beyond the old equation of simply working for money.

Just as managers have a major impact on the intrinsic motivation of their staff's jobs, so they have a direct role in encouraging and maintaining social cohesion at work.

Changing motivation

A moment's thought tells us that the potency of the factors that motivate us will vary between people and over time. A sudden and unexpected need to generate more income might persuade somebody to focus on economic issues at the expense of intrinsic and social ones. This could result in them looking for a better-paid job even though they may leave behind a valued network of work colleagues. Also, it seems that for many people the first half of their working life is characterised by the need for achievement and proving themselves within their chosen profession. Later in life, questions of meaning and purpose in life often become more prominent. Where this is true, people may choose roles that satisfy a need to feel useful in society even when this may entail economic sacrifices.

We mentioned earlier the good and bad news about motivation. Money is a short-term motivator that might affect *where* we work and *why* we might change job, but, by and large, team managers do not determine levels of pay. Intrinsic and social motivations affect how we perform and these are the ones that the local manager *can* and must influence.

Here are some suggestions as to *how* you as a manager can increase the intrinsic and social factors in your staff's day-to-day work.

➤ Take a moment to consider the jobs your team do. What scope is there for each person to extract social or intrinsic motivation from their job? What could you do to increase this scope?

➤ Be aware of emerging friendships and look for opportunities to place people together for both enjoyable and challenging tasks.

➤ If cliques emerge ask the members to reflect on the impact their exclusiveness might have on the team.

➤ Find out what interests the person and ask them to suggest ways in which their job can be enhanced to accommodate some of these interests – the appraisal discussion is ideal for this (*see* below).

➤ Genuinely thank staff for their efforts, not in a sweeping statement to all at the end of a shift, but in a one to one conversation highlighting specifics.

➤ Catch people doing things right and tell them straightaway.

➤ Identify those who are naturally good instructors and teachers and invite them to 'adopt' new employees.

➤ Let people know you trust them, and that your absence on other business is an expression of that trust, not a sign of disinterest.

➤ Ask your staff how they would prefer to be managed, and then act on their response!

Appraisal

A basic requirement for almost all people at work is an answer to the question, *'How am I doing?'*.

Different organisations have different names to describe the process of regularly meeting staff to discuss prior performance and prepare for the next few months: appraisal, personal development review (PDR), individual performance review (IPR), supervision, annual review. In some client organisations there is a move to capture the discussion and the outcomes of such discussions electronically, with the result that the letter 'e' prefaces many of the labels.

Regardless of the label, in our discussion with clients we have discovered a number of unspoken assumptions about the process of appraisal. These are:

➤ the expectation that the process is always annual (or at other fixed periods)

➤ that all staff are 'appraised' at the same time of year or within a short fixed timescale

➤ that all staff are allocated the same time slot for their session

➤ an expectation that appraisal is organised *and* led by the manager

➤ an acceptance that the meeting will take place in the manager's office, will probably be interrupted and is likely to be postponed at short notice if the manager is 'called away'.

These assumptions combine to produce low employee opinions as to the humanity of the process, their employer's commitment and the overall value.

Michael West (*see* Chapter 1) has discovered that positive appraisal is a significant component of effective organisations, and our own empirical research suggests that a person's experience of appraisal (either positive or negative) has a major impact on their sense of feeling valued – and consequently their willingness to offer more to that organisation.

> On many of our programmes we ask participants how long it has been since their last appraisal. At the time of writing this book, the current record is 12 years. In the Introduction we discussed the need people have to know how they are doing, coupled with the reluctance of some managers to sit down with a colleague and answer that question. For anyone to have to work for 12 years without ever having a chance to sit down and discuss their performance is both a waste of that person's potential to do better and a major challenge to that organisation's espoused belief that it values its staff.

So how do you create the right environment for the appraisal discussion to take place and be constructive for both parties? It doesn't take exceptional communication skills, powerful oratory or devastating wit. In fact we would describe appraisal as simply a conversation with a purpose. This requires a genuine commitment to your staff and their development as evidenced by your willingness to spend time and effort meeting their needs.

Purpose

The primary purpose of appraisal is to encourage dialogue about a person's prior, current and future performance, so that good practice is recognised and maintained, and areas for improvement are supported and addressed. It is a tool for development, not discipline.

The ingredients of appraisal

➤ A culture of trust and respect throughout the organisation, so that the activity is undertaken openly and without suspicion.

➤ Clarity of roles, both in the job and in the discussion, so that no one is confused as to what is expected from the job and the exchange of views.

➤ Prior agreement on any objectives being reviewed and the criteria to be used, to prevent accusations of the goalposts being moved.

➤ skilled appraiser, i.e. someone who knows the members of staff, knows how to conduct a discussion and who can give sensitive and constructive feedback.

➤ receptive appraisee, i.e. someone who wants to be there, sees the process as helpful and trusts the intentions of the manager.

➤ No surprises for either side; in other words, nothing introduced that has not already been raised at the time it happened.

➤ Emphasis on praise; not lies or false praise, but genuine recognition of good work.

➤ Self-reflection, where both parties do some thinking before the discussion itself.

➤ Space, and as much time as the the appraisee wants or needs.

Preparation is vital if the appraisal discussion is to contain these elements, and here are some pointers to effective preparation.

➤ **Give good notice of the date and time of the session, and its purpose.** Why not allow the appraisee to choose the date and time as this can reduce the sense of appraisal being *done to* the person? Also why not ask them where might be a good place? After all, whose meeting is it?

➤ **Invite the appraisee to come prepared with the following.**
   — Their views on their own performance over the past period, both in terms of their formal objectives and their personal contribution. We often find that, given the opportunity, people are harder on themselves than an appraiser would be.
   — Their ideas on objectives for the coming period.
   — Their thoughts on development needs connected with these objectives.

➤ **Gather your thoughts and evidence on the same three areas.**

➤ **Remember, no surprises.** Your own perceptions are useful evidence but try to add harder data if available. Make sure any poor performance areas can be corroborated by others and do not introduce anything that has not already been highlighted at the time it happened. *Never* 'store up' issues to raise at the next appraisal.

The discussion itself has to be the product of the wishes and personalities of the two people involved. Do not be tempted to use exactly the same format for each person in order to achieve 'consistency'. This is a false economy and sends the signal to staff that they are merely part of a 'sheep dipping' exercise.

On a recent programme we heard of an organisation where the managers were under pressure to get the outstanding appraisals carried out as soon as possible and, at the same time, ensure that the new computerised record system was completed. This combination of time pressures and new systems led to a plan to 'give everyone five minutes'. We will leave it to your imagination to work out what the staff involved thought of the process and their likely attitude towards the next year's round of appraisals.

Environment

Choose a place that allows for open discussion. We have appraised staff in offices, over a coffee in Starbucks and during a stroll around a lake. If you and the appraisee would feel more comfortable 'on the premises' you might still look for an area away from the immediate work environment. Some ward managers we know of agree to use each other's ward meeting rooms to give that sense of distance and privacy. Wherever you agree to meet, desks usually imply a formal status barrier, so it might be less threatening if you come out and sit alongside the appraisee. However, if the desk is part of your style and you are famous for it, it could be more discomforting if you did come out from behind it. The appraisee might suspect some amateur psychology at work and be less open as a result. Remember, no surprises.

Time

If you want to send a negative message to an appraisee, tell them their time is up halfway through the discussion. Give at least an hour, preferably two, and have something useful up your sleeve to do if the session finishes early. If you say, *'We have as long as we need'*, and you mean it, you will send a powerful signal of your commitment. Never schedule several sessions for the same morning or afternoon, and try to get agreement from your managers for the whole process to be carried out over a broad timescale so that staff do not feel processed by a corporate agenda.

The discussion

You will be expected to set the scene so take light control at the start. It will put the appraisee on edge if you just sit back at the start and say 'so what shall we talk about' in an attempt to make the session informal. Use *we* and *us*, as in, 'Would it be helpful for us to go through the last year/month/quarter?', and provide a structure. Using the three preparation points mentioned earlier might be helpful.

➤ Prior performance.
➤ New objectives.
➤ Support required.

Having set the scene and the structure, invite the appraisee to make the first judgement about either general performance or a specific objective. Some appraisers like to start with an overview while others like to get straight into the first objective. Both approaches are valid, but it gets the session off on the right note if the *appraisee* has the first shot. This reinforces self-reflection, and gives you clues as to whether their degree of self-awareness is high or low. Armed with this information, you can then introduce your feedback and assessment in an appropriate way.

Once the appraisee has had their say, you will be expected to respond, either in support of the self-assessment or to qualify it from your own perspective. Avoid challenging the individual on their right to have their own view if it conflicts with your own. A better strategy would be to acknowledge the person's view, add your own and invite both of you to discuss the reasons for the difference. Saying *'I can't see how you could possibly see that as a success!'* simply promotes an argument about the person not the issue.

Although appraisal is used in some organisations for assessing eligibility for additional financial rewards, the discussion itself is more fruitful if it concentrates on the reasons for successes and failures, and ways of promoting or avoiding these in the future.

Appraisal is *developmental* not disciplinary. The time for 'penalising' behaviour is not during appraisal. Similarly, humiliation and destroyed confidence, however accidental, are poor outcomes from the appraisal process.

Wherever possible tackle problem areas by referring to earlier discussions you might have had with the person. It is unacceptable for the appraisee to be informed for the first time of your dissatisfaction months after an incident took place. Being able to refer to the fact that *'we talked about this at the time but it doesn't seem to have improved'* is more powerful than throwing surprises or long-forgotten issues into the discussion. This does, of course, presuppose that there were regular prior discussions with staff and that this formal appraisal is not the person's sole contact with their manager!

Finish on three positives.

1   The first is a summary of the positive parts of the appraisal content.
2   The second is a positive action plan for addressing any personal or technical development issues raised – do not rake over the coals, simply concentrate on what is going to happen now.
3   The third is a positive statement about the session itself, its value to the person, its value to you and the need to keep in touch.

Record the outcomes and actions, communicate these to the appraisee in a letter or form acceptable to your organisation, and ask for their acceptance of the findings and the action plan.

With the increase in computerisation of appraisal records comes a new challenge. How do you keep the dialogue going and the whole process feeling personal when one or both of you are looking at a computer screen? Even more challenging to your attempts to create the right atmosphere is having the conversation driven by the next section of the e-record. It's a bit like going to see your doctor or lawyer but finding his or her computer screen in the way. Our advice is don't try! Although we appear to be advocating taking more time, try to have the first part of the discussion as free flowing as possible and once you have both agreed the main points, use the second half, or a separate short meeting, to fill in the forms. By all means also use the forms to guide the preparation stage so that both parties are aware of the information required, but please, do not try to have the conversation and enter data at the same time. You will be distracted and the member of staff will know exactly what their organisation thinks of them. The result will almost certainly be unsatisfactory for both parties. Worse still, the coffee-room conversation between that member of staff and the next person to be appraised will not give that person much confidence.

There are a number of strategies that can be employed when having to raise areas of criticism, but again remember, no surprises. Do not bring up anything that has not already been discussed at the time it occurred. Points to remember are listed below.

➤ **Positive/negative/positive.** Start with a positive item, then raise the negative as something which is undoing or undermining the good work rather than as simply a mistake, and then finish with another positive. This framework can be used for the whole meeting as well as a particular item of feedback.

➤ **Describe the behaviour or the issue, not the person.** Saying 'You are lazy' is both rude and unhelpful. 'You do seem to take time finishing some of the important stuff – do you know what causes this?' is less personally threatening and encourages self-reflection.

➤ **Try to avoid using the word 'why'.** This is easier to write about than to comply with for most of us, but that small word can be incredibly threatening and can cause people to become defensive. '*What was your thinking behind that idea?*' displays more of a genuine attempt to understand, whereas '*Why did you do that?*' can easily be taken to mean that you would do it differently, i.e. right, and they did it wrong.

➤ **Be realistic.** If your assessment of their self-awareness shows them to be reluctant or incapable of picking up subtle messages, you still have an obligation to give it to them straight, and live with the consequences of any ensuing argument or emotion. However, the above strategies can prevent such tension from becoming the norm.

General principles for giving feedback

Whether in the middle of appraisal or during other informal discussions, you will occasionally be in a position where some honest feedback would be helpful. Here are some guiding principles.

➤ **Feedback should be descriptive rather than evaluative or judgemental.** In other words it should describe what you saw, heard or felt. It should not be accompanied by analysis or judgement. You might choose to say '*When you chaired that meeting, I observed you commenting on each item before giving others the chance to speak. Did you notice that and what are your reflections on how it went?*' You should not say '*Your chairing was overbearing and disempowered everyone else there*'.

➤ **Feedback should be solicited not imposed.** This means ensuring that the person is ready for feedback and ideally has actively wanted your observations.

Just getting something off your chest may meet your needs but is very unlikely to meet the other person's needs and could well lead to defensiveness and an argument.

➤ **Feedback should be referenced on issues, not generalisations of behaviour or personality.** Again, the key is to be specific and descriptive. *'When we last discussed this matter, I felt overwhelmed by your enthusiasm for the idea and ended up agreeing rather than introducing my own idea'* is more likely to produce a constructive dialogue than *'You are a bit of a bully and always want your own way'*, even if the latter is said with a smile on your face.

➤ **Feedback should be focused on something the recipient can do something about.** Tall people are unable to make themselves smaller just to stop themselves being a bit intimidating to shorter people. People who have a neutral face are unlikely to change their features. Happy people are happy for a reason, and should not be made to change. Therefore make sure that what you are feeding back is something that, a) they can work on changing, and b) you are prepared to help them with.

Personal development planning

As with appraisal, personal development planning is becoming increasingly pro ceduralised. By this we mean that computerised forms are fast becoming the way personal development ideas are expressed and captured. We are not against this in principle because we recognise that it allows the aggregation of skills, competencies, gaps and interests by organisations that can then resource their HR and training func- tions to meet those needs. If we have an unease it is that these electronic records can inadvertently depersonalise the process and lead to a situation where the person has to 'fit the template' rather than the other way round. As long as the forms and the templates are seen as tools to support and record planning, and not as limits to that thinking, we are content, and this next section looks at different ways of undertak- ing this critical task.

General Dwight David Eisenhower, leader of the Allied invasion of Europe during World War II and later the 34th US President, offered this thought on the process of planning: *'In preparing for battle, I have always found that plans are useless but planning is indispensable'*[1].

Eisenhower's point is that while the finished article, the plan, is almost certain to be overtaken by events, the process of planning is where the quality thinking and the insights emerge. The act of gathering opinions and facts, thinking them through, being challenged, etc. all of these are indispensable but the final plan is at best temporary.

We adopt this approach in the way we work with clients in personal development planning. The process of thinking through ideas, options and ideals is where the value lies. Of course, there needs to be some action that follows and turning it into a document will be helpful in many cases. However, unless the planning is sound the plan will be worthless and will lack any real ownership.

So, without undermining the need of organisations to capture consistent information on the development needs of their staff, here is our approach to PDP (personal development planning) that tends to produce real commitment to change.

We are going to start with you. Of course you could just read this section and then move on to the rest of the book but if you want to think about your own personal development, set aside about 30 minutes to go through the following exercise. Personal experience will then help you reflect on the uses and benefits of this approach with your own staff!

PDP in 30 minutes!

Do not self-edit or overthink your answers to the following questions. Just jot down whatever comes to you. No one else will see it and you can always revisit your thinking afterwards. Also, despite the temptation to read ahead, try to just stick to the question in front of you, otherwise you will start to limit your creativity.

First, take a sheet of A4 paper and divide it into five sections (this is not rocket science but if you draw four horizontal lines across the page equally spaced down the sheet you will magically produce five sections!).

In the first section, note your initial responses to these questions in turn:
➤ Where am I in my development as a manager?
➤ What are my biggest work challenges/objectives?
➤ To what extent am I living out my life goals?

In the second section, note your responses to these questions in turn:
➤ How would I like things to be in my work?
➤ What do I most need to learn to do differently?
➤ What life goals do I most want to achieve?

In the third section, note your responses to these questions in turn:
➤ In the next 12 months, what actions/processes would help me change my practice as a manager?
➤ In the next 12 months, what could I do to move nearer to my life goals?

In the fourth section, note down your response to this question:
➤ Who's help and support might I need to achieve these things?

In the final section, note down:
➤ The next three things I need to do to begin to turn the plan into reality.

Before we give you some of our thoughts on that process, and its challenges, take a moment to step back and reflect. What has that exercise revealed or confirmed for you? Were any parts more difficult or challenging than others and why might that be? How different was it from previous PDP exercises? Did doing it quickly allow you to put down what you really think or did it feel rushed and superficial?

In our work with managers we find that this approach creates more depth and reflection than participants have experienced before. The fusion of work challenges and life goals is a surprise to some but remember that the whole person comes to work and the whole person takes their experiences back home with them. For some, the exercise gently prods them to do what they have always wanted to but never taken seriously. Others find that they have been working to please others rather than meet their own needs. For a couple of participants the exercise actually confirmed that the job they were doing was not what they really wanted and they subsequently changed careers.

Obviously we make no hard and fast promises for this exercise. However, we constantly find that, for the first time in a long time, it puts the person right at the centre of their thinking and encourages a holistic view of their development. It promotes taking responsibility for one's own development whilst, interestingly, strengthening the relationship between staff and employer.

Now that you have experienced the process, here is a question for you. Could you make the same opportunity for reflection and planning available to your staff and what impact might it have on their motivation, empowerment and relationship with you?

Go ahead, try it out. If nothing else you will gain additional insights into your staff, insights that you can then incorporate into how you then motivate and manage them in the future. Some managers have used the whole tool whereas others have weaved some of the questions into the appraisal conversation. Think about each member of staff as an individual – what might work best for them?

Tackling poor performance

So far we have looked at the preparation for, and stewardship of, an appraisal discussion and given you a model to support thinking about your own, and your staff's development. However, poor performance can crop up at any time and we have already mentioned that the appraisal discussion is not the place to bring up such issues for the first time. For many new managers, tackling dips in performance is the least enjoyable part of their role, particularly because it may involve awkward discussions with their friends and workmates (if the manager was promoted from within the team).

In all probability your current organisation will have carefully considered policies for handling performance issues and it is vital that you are guided by those at all times. In this book we will be looking at some of the principles that should under-pin your *personal* response to those staff who are not doing as well as expected, and some of the interpersonal *behaviours* that will help you through what can be a difficult and emotional time.

The first thing to say about any morally defensible approach to managing performance is that its aims should be *prevention, support and remedy*. If you are working for an organisation that uses its performance management system for purposes of punishment, retribution or entrapment, then perhaps you need to find another employer!

We make a distinction between performance management and disciplinary action. The latter is designed to correct personal behaviour that is unacceptable and damaging to the organisation and its clients. If behaviour does not change then punitive measures, ultimately including dismissal, are perfectly reasonable as long as they are handled professionally and legally. Managing poor performance is based on the assumption that the person is not wilfully behaving in a malicious way and that other factors are currently causing their level of performance to be less than required by the standards of the job or less than was previously delivered. In short, the goal of tackling poor performance should be a return to form!

Poor performance can have a number of causes and the following list is illustrative rather than exhaustive.

➤ Lack of training or instruction.
➤ Underlying relationship issues with clients or other members of staff.
➤ Non-work-related issues impacting on work.
➤ Loss of confidence.
➤ Ignorance as to the required standards.
➤ Lack of self-awareness.
➤ Different expectations between employers.

There are five principles that should guide both an organisation's corporate approach to managing performance and the day-to-day behaviour of individual managers towards their staff. If you are currently employed, take a look at your employer's policy handbook and you should find evidence of these five foundation blocks.

TABLE 2.1 Five principles for managing performance

Clarity	The line manager should ensure that there is a clear and explicit common understanding with all staff as to their role and expected standards of performance. Managers and supervisors should ensure that the general performance, standards and attendance of staff are monitored as a matter of routine. This should allow them to identify and resolve problems at an early stage through informal methods, and to ensure that consistent standards and expectations are being applied to all employees within the group.
Uniqueness	Whilst following a consistent approach and applying consistent criteria, each case should be examined and treated on its merits and according to individual circumstances.
Dialogue	The employee should have been given a chance to explain the reasons for the problem, and then given reasonable opportunity and support to improve their performance. There should be a clear common understanding of the shortfalls in performance, the improvements required, and the timescale allowed for those improvements to be demonstrated.
Agreement	There should be a clear common understanding of any steps that the manager has agreed to take in order to support and assist the employee to achieve the improvements required, and to monitor progress and provide feedback in the meantime.
Documentation	All formal discussions and arrangements with the employee under these guidelines should be fully documented, together with any evidence of the performance shortfall, with copies made available to the employee (and, if requested, to their representative). This is so the employer can subsequently demonstrate at appeal or to any third party that they have taken reasonable steps to act fairly and reasonably under the circumstances of the case.

As you read those principles it would be difficult to find fault with any of them or to suggest that they might not always apply. That is the hallmark of a good principle! However, principles are easy to write down and they sound worthy. But what do you need to do if you find yourself actually having to have the conversation with a member of the team who seems not to be coping?

Six tactics will help you here.

TABLE 2.2 Six tactics for successful discussions with employees

Timing	Get in quickly and ask 'What is happening?', or 'Is there a problem?' The key to effective management of performance is timeliness. Remember you are not collecting incriminating evidence, you are simply seeing someone in difficulty, or hearing reports of someone in difficulty, and your first response should be to offer help. Many managers run into problems when the time gap between the problem first occuring and the discussion is so large that either no one can confidently recall events, or the employee is reasonably entitled to believe that what they have been doing has been accepted by the employer.
	Longer-term monitoring may be acceptable if early discussions have not led to any improvement and there appears to be a deliberate intention to act inappropriately, but otherwise step in early and ask if everything is okay. Do not summon people to the office, or set up a formal appointment for a few days time; these approaches simply
Setting	The discussion should be conducted in a confidential setting but using an informal, counselling style to discuss openly the performance problems and any underlying causes. The manager should ask relevant open questions relating to work performance; intrusive or personal matters relating to the employee's medical or domestic circumstances should not be raised unless introduced by the employee, although you should imply that those areas can be mentioned if the person wishes.
Analysing the 'gap'	Clearly state, and restate if needed, the standards and expectations of performance in the role, referring where appropriate to job descriptions, standing instructions and suchlike. This may require the establishment of a clear work programme, with proper supervision and adequate guidance and monitoring.
	Be precise and emotion-free about the shortfalls in performance, the underlying reasons for these and the timescales agreed for the necessary improvements to be made. It is important that the employee agrees that the reasons for the problems have been fully discussed and supports the proposed solutions, otherwise they may continually raise new issues at later stages that they claim were not properly considered.
	Offer support from yourself and the wider organisation, for example on-the-job training or formal instruction, in order to achieve required standards, but do not leave the employee with the impression that others will do everything and they have no part to play.
	(If the discussion is not the first time the issue has been raised and there is the risk of a pattern of non-compliance emerging, then it may be appropriate to include the following.)
	Be clear and, again, *emotion-free*, about the consequences of failing to achieve the required standards in the timescale and sustain them thereafter. These could range from withholding of increments to redeployment, downgrading or dismissal.
	In some cases the employee may suggest that personal or domestic circumstances outside work may be affecting their performance at work, and from a welfare point of view the employer will fully accept that staff may need support and understanding

(continued)

during periods of personal difficulty before they can return to normal standards of performance. However, such reasons do not discharge them from their long-term contractual responsibilities at work, and you must be satisfied that their problems are short term and can be overcome – or, if related to a long-term disability, can be overcome by a reasonable adjustment. Such cases should be referred through HR so that specialist support and advice can be obtained.

Focus Again, the aim of such support will be to support the employee towards returning to the achievement of normal standards of performance as soon as possible, and to obtain a professional prognosis of likely timescales for this, advice on any restrictions on duties or hours which should be observed in the interim, and so forth.

Timescales Timescales, allowed for the necessary improvements in performance to take place, must be reasonable, and take into account the natural length of the work cycle where the problem has occurred as well as any time required for training. For example, issues such as timekeeping or attendance should be capable of improvement over relatively short periods, but the improvements in the production of monthly statistics may take some time to show through.

Review Having agreed and documented the targets and measures for improvement it is essential that these be followed through, that regular monitoring and feedback takes place throughout the review period and that the manager ensures delivery of any measures promised by way of documentation, guidance or training to assist the employee.

The relationship between management and staff

Hopefully you will be aware by now that to manage individuals successfully you need to adopt an individual approach to each one. Management styles may have attractive titles and the desire to seek out your default style is extremely seductive. However, the real world does not always operate the way your chosen style would like and the simple fact is that if you approach people-management issues in the same way every time, you will be like a clock that has stopped – you will be right twice a day! The rest of the time you will simply fail to meet the needs of the member of staff in front of you.

A more productive way of thinking about the managerial relationship is to consider the phrase *situational leadership*. Rather like the famous wood-stain advertisement, it does exactly what it says on the tin. It encourages managers to analyse the situation in front of them (which includes both the task to be done and the person affected) and then adopt the most appropriate style of leadership behaviour. Sounds simple and obvious doesn't it? However, it also requires managers to do the antithesis of what most corporate organisations want – behave inconsistently.

Some years ago, a worldwide research study was undertaken by Paul Hersey and Kenneth H Blanchard (*Management of Organizational Behavior: utilizing human resources.* Englewood Cliffs, NJ: Prentice-Hall; 1988) into what people saw as effective leadership

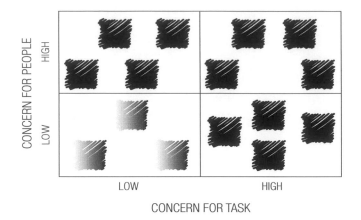

FIGURE 2.1 Concern for people versus concern for task I

and who typified a good leader. The researchers' initial hypothesis was that people would comment on a leader's ability to give equal weight to the task at hand (the problem or issue) and the needs of the people. They therefore borrowed an existing model showing the relationship between those two factors. When they plotted the results they found a completely random distribution, as shown in Figure 2.1.

It seemed strange that some people could describe some 'good' leaders as those with seemingly little regard for either the task or the people involved, but this gave Hersey and Blanchard the clue. Good leadership is determined by the led, and may not be an innate characteristic of the leader. It seems that, depending upon the situation that people find themselves in and their current state of need, different styles of leadership are more appropriate and staff recognise this intuitively.

When people are new to a task, lacking in confidence, unsure of what they can and cannot do, what they often need is *directing* and *telling*, no nonsense, and no room for error.

As they become more aware of their surroundings, and get some feedback as to what they can and cannot do, they tend to need more of a *coaching* style of management and leadership, where they are given some responsibility while being gently steered towards particular ways of operating.

As their competence and confidence steadily improves, they may respond best to a more *supportive* style of leadership, one that puts them in control but provides back-up as and when they require it.

Once people become competent and comfortable in their work and situation, the most appropriate way of handling them could be to leave them alone, to *delegate* the work and the way in which it is done, and stop meddling.

Let us put those different styles on the same grid (Figure 2.2).

Now those seemingly random results make sense. The four styles of leadership

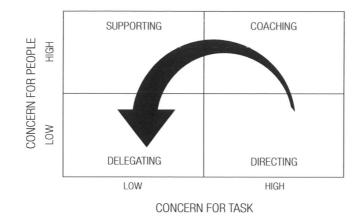

FIGURE 2.2 Concern for people versus concern for task II

are proper responses to the situations in which people find themselves, and they allow leaders to be more or less concerned with task/people based on those situations.

The arrow suggests that leaders are constantly wishing to move staff to the next, less reliant, level of leadership style, although we are slightly concerned that this may be unrealistic for those staff who simply do not want to reach the stage of self-management. It also implies that there is only one direction of travel, whereas in real life people have crises of confidence and may respond to a temporary increase in leadership control and direction.

We find this approach to leadership is well received by managers and students alike and seems to strike a chord with new managerial recruits. However, situational leadership does not just happen, regardless of the acceptance of the model. Good situational leaders seem to be those who can:

➤ create an environment and culture where people are encouraged to articulate what they need in the way of managing and leading, without feeling judged or pilloried
➤ pick up the clues that staff send out about those needs, by being around, being interested and being available
➤ adapt their own personal style to meet the needs of the situation that exists at that time, and, most importantly
➤ live with the potential criticism that they are being inconsistent in their treatment of others.

How do you rate yourself against these four characteristics?

Unless leaders act in this flexible, situational way, they risk having only one style, the one that is more comfortable to them and which they try to use in most situations, perhaps in an attempt to be consistent and honourable. However, a one-size-fits-all style is unlikely to release the potential of your staff, and could even do damage to some.

THE PROS AND CONS OF HAVING AN INFLEXIBLE LEADERSHIP STYLE

As a fresh faced 20-year-old, I worked in a junior clerical role. The supervisor was a middle-aged lady who spent most of her spare time organising girl guides. She was a no-nonsense, task-focused manager who was always explicit about what she wanted done. She was directive and clear, and gave immediate feedback on performance. I always thought of her as a good boss but was puzzled at the time by her unpopularity with the other staff, who were all mature ladies with many years experience.

Situational leadership sheds some light on this. For a young man in his first 'proper' job, this directive style was ideal. I needed to be told what to do and where to go, and because I left after 8 months I never outgrew it. But for the other staff, who knew their jobs and were experienced, this constantly directing style must have been patronising and frustrating. (AP)

If you prefer telling and directing (and there is nothing inherently wrong with such an approach) there are times when you will be holding people back and preventing them from developing. Similarly, if you prefer to adopt more of a laid-back and supportive style, there will be times when you will leave people vulnerable and unsure. At its most extreme this hands-off approach can leave people feeling abandoned and reluctant to take responsibility in the future. Of course there will be some who do not wish to develop to the point of being totally self-sufficient and you should guard against pushing them along the big arrow in the diagram. Some voluntary staff, in particular, may have chosen such work because it does not require major responsibilities and they may resent a dogmatic system of 'weaning them off' appropriate management support.

Again, the key is to be sensitive to the different needs of clients, staff, other managers, etc. and choose an approach that meets those needs. To do otherwise is to provide a poor return for the trust that such people put in those who manage them.

Finally in this chapter about the manager's relationship with staff, we introduce some psychology. However, in line with the theme of the whole book we will keep it simple and practical.

It's time to be honest. Are there some people in your life or workplace with whom you keep getting into a repeating pattern of behaviour? You do or say something to them, they respond a particular way, which in turn reinforces your stance, which you restate, and round and round you go? Often the spectators are all too aware of this destructive cycle whereas the participants are too busy 'being themselves' and both feel completely justified in their behaviour.

One way of both explaining and guarding against these self-maintaining patterns is the study of transactional analysis or TA. Developed by Eric Berne (*Games People Play – the psychology of human relationships*. London: Penguin, 1964), it is a highly complex view of human interactions but in this book we are concentrating on one just type of dialogue.

TA suggests that each person in a relationship/conversation has the choice of three general behavioural states, labelled *parental, adult* or *childlike*. Each has sub-divisions but here are the edited highlights.

➤ *Parental* mode involves accessing our memories of being parented and acting in a way that takes control, manages risk, assumes the 'moral high ground', tells rather than suggests and judges rather than stays neutral. It can be loving as well as controlling but the core message is 'I know best'.

➤ *Adult* mode involves a mature view of equality and a desire for a mutual search for progress and solutions. It comes from our experience of living alongside others who also have needs and rights.

➤ *Childlike* mode involves accessing memories of being a child and being subject to parental behaviour. It is typified by avoiding responsibility, withdrawing under criticism, being spontaneous, experimenting, challenging authority and pushing boundaries, and by having fun.

You would think that each party has free choice of their state or mode when having a conversation. In practice we observe that the choice exercised by the first person to speak tends to 'condition' the response of the other person, leading to a situation where the subsequent behaviour of each party simply reinforces and amplifies the reaction of the other. We find that onlookers often spot this developing loop and can usually predict how the conversation is going to escalate, but the protagonists seem both blind to it and hell-bent on 'winning' the argument by cranking up their own behaviour.

The most obvious example of this sort of behaviour is the manager tackling a member of staff using a somewhat parental stance.

Manager	Look here, what do you think you are doing? How many times have I told you not to speak to people that way? (Parental stance)
Staff member	I'm overworked, you are never around to support me, what the hell do you expect for £X per hour? I don't know why I stay here! (Childlike stance)
Manager	Don't speak to me like that. We have professional standards here and you are being unprofessional. You've been like this since you started.

> If you don't change your ways things will get serious! (Reinforced parental stance)
>
> Staff member   You can't threaten me; I'm off to see the union. This is a lousy place to work and anyone would be mad to work for you. (Reinforced childlike stance)

What is significant about this sort of exchange is that each person's comments simply confirm the other person's view that they were right to take the stance they did. We once heard a 'parental' manager describe her staff as 'a bunch of kids who need constant supervision otherwise the place would fall apart', blissfully unaware that her parental attitude was creating the very childlike behaviours she was then having to address.

> We have observed that staff will often use childlike behaviour when asking for help with IT issues. Staff who are normally assertive and confident use every childlike trick in the book in the hope that the IT specialist will come and fix their problem. Bambi eyes, head on one side and a wheedling tone of voice are all brought into play as the staff member tries to get the specialist to come, and, like a parent, make the problem go away.

It is important to remember that the manager is just as capable of coming across in childlike mode, which leads the staff member to become parental, and the manager adopts even more extreme childlike behaviour, and again the destructive pattern is set.

The key to avoiding or rescuing these situations is self-awareness. The manager must be able to spot the trigger words and situations that lead them into parental or childlike behaviours and adopt the third stance – that of adult. Remember adult behaviour involves mutual trust and respect, a desire for dialogue and collaboration. We have found that if one party adopts an adult stance from the start of a conversation it is difficult for the other person to maintain the unhelpful parental or childlike behaviours, because there is nothing to feed off or kick against. Over time, the other person will adopt their own adult stance either because it seems the only way to make progress, or because the reasonableness of the first person defuses the situation.

Two real life case studies will illustrate this point.

> Two managers were facing the same problem – staff appraisals having to be competed within a short timescale at a time when overtime had been stopped, staff sickness was high and all teams were struggling to cope.

Manager A took the stance of feeling so unsupported and overwhelmed that she made it clear that she would not comply, would not notify anyone she was not complying, and announced, *'Lets see what happens when they find out – but it is not my problem now.'* This was highly childlike behaviour and it was almost inevitable that this person's manager, once they found out, would be hostile, controlling and extremely parental. Manager A would, in turn, feel abused and even if she did finally comply it would be with huge reluctance and sulking (reinforced childlike behaviour). Imagine how her staff would feel when the appraisals finally took place.

Facing the same issue, **Manager B** thought the matter through, developed a workable alternative proposal, rang her manager and said, *'I am having difficulties meeting this target because of X. However if you give me an extra two weeks I can get the appraisals done, keep the staff on board, and get another key issue moved forward. Does this sound okay to you?'* In this example, the senior manager not only said yes but also thanked Manager B for taking the trouble to ring rather than send an email.

Adult behaviour by Manager B produced adult behaviour by the senior manager, and the relationship between the two would almost certainly prosper in the future. In contrast, Manager A would quickly be labelled as difficult by the management regime (and by her staff).

If you can recognise times when your approach to staff has been parental or childlike, and you want things to be different, the simple but vital message is . . . the manager must blink first!

These examples of TA at work are a powerful reminder to all of us that it is easy to drop into a particular behavioural stance, and there will be many times when we are quite justified in feeling as we do. The point is that the manager has to take responsibility for changing their behaviour first. You simply cannot afford to wait for some one to 'come to their senses'. Phrases like *'when they start acting like adults I will treat them like adults'* sound rational but the manager will be waiting a very long time! Remember you are a role model for your staff. If they see you acting bossy or petulant they will lose respect for you and will almost unconsciously start to behave in the opposite ways. These loops of behaviour are easy to fall into, and hard for the protagonists to spot. For the self-aware manager, however, they are relatively easy to change by adopting adult-to-adult behaviours.

The following list contains some sample questions that you can use during a conversation to demonstrate adult behaviour and in turn elicit an adult response. If you customise these and incorporate them into conversations with your staff, you will find that even difficult characters will begin to engage in adult behaviour in return. It may not work immediately with everyone (after all you may be trying to change several years of reinforcing loops) but persevere and you will see results.

➤ How do you want to handle this?

➤ When would be a good time?

➤ How much information do you want at this stage?

➤ Who should I speak to?

➤ How do you see this problem?

➤ How much time do we have?

➤ What should I take into account when approaching this person/task?

➤ What would help to move this forward?

The following phrases can also help when you need to establish rapport in situations that could be challenging or sensitive.

➤ I don't know about you but there are times when I feel uneasy about/am confused by your . . .

➤ I am quite clear on what is required by when, etc. You need to know that one of the factors that may compromise this project is X and I would value your thoughts in how *we* might tackle it.

➤ Please clarify exactly what your expectations are of me/my team – without this we may waste considerable time and effort.

➤ Before we get stuck in, would it be helpful to go over how project X worked out, particularly how the two teams worked together, so we don't make the same mistakes again?

➤ Can I start by making clear our opportunities and constraints? We can do A by September at current staffing/workloads. But we can do B by August if project X is deferred until October. How would those two scenarios impact on you?

Hopefully you can see that the common thread running through all those phrases is a genuine desire to collaborate and recognise the other person's needs/interests in the situation. Simply forcing one view over another is a recipe for another destructive loop!

CONCLUSION

Most people simply resent being treated as just one of the crowd. Effective managers are those who are able to do more than simply accept that people are different – they actively incorporate a desire to treat people uniquely into their day-to-day practice. Picking up the themes of this chapter, we are motivated by different stimuli; we have different expectations and needs of the appraisal process; our performance dips and recovers for different reasons; our personal development aspirations are unique; and we respond to different styles of leadership at different times in our career and for different tasks. Finally, we wish to be treated as adults, not parents or children.

Thoughtful management involves truly understanding the wants and needs of our staff and then working with each one uniquely to help them give their best. Moreover, it requires a huge dollop of trust – a belief that most staff come to work wanting to do a good job and all they need is support from their manager in order to do so.

An author who has inspired and influenced much of our management development practice over recent years is Ricardo Semler, a Brazilian businessman who has gone further than most in introducing genuine empowerment and democracy in his company, Semco. We conclude this chapter with a comment from his book, *Maverick*,[2] that pretty much sums up the way most people would like to be managed but which, sadly, very few actually experience.

> *We simply do not believe that our employees have an interest in coming in late, leaving early and doing as little as possible for as much money as their union can wheedle out of us . . . We trust them. We don't make our employees ask permission to go to the bathroom, or have security guards search them as they leave for the day. We get out of their way and let them do their job.*

Do you agree, and can you create that environment for your team?

As a footnote it is interesting that Semler also has an approach to staff development which can be summed up as 'we will find you something you are good at!'. Many other organisations have the opposite approach of locking people into jobs they struggle to do, by identifying their weaknesses and trying to fix them. If you want an example of a UK version of Semler's approach, read Richard Branson's books on his approach to recognising talent.

REFERENCES

1 Wheatley M, Kellner-Rogers M. *A Simpler Way*. San Francisco: Berret Koehler; 1996.
2 Semler R. *Maverick*. London: Arrow Books; 1994.

CHAPTER 3

Leading change

All management is change management. Maybe in some sepia-tinted industrial past managers were paid to keep things ticking over, but in today's workplace all managers are expected to implement or instigate change more or less continually. And rightly so. If better ways can be found to heal patients, run airlines or deliver parcels we should introduce them.

It is a testament to good sense and good managers that so much change is managed with so little fuss. Every day, in thousands of organisations, new staff are trained, absent staff covered for, unexpected demands coped with and good ideas tried out. Where change goes well it is either unnoticed or called improvement rather than change. It is the mismanaged change that catches our attention. At boardroom level this often takes the shape of a reorganisation or merger that fails to bring the promised benefits. At team-leader level, the focus of this book, it might be attempts by the team leader to improve the way the team works that meet with resistance, or new 'improved' systems that paradoxically lead to more work or lowered standards. But surely, such failures are the exception rather than the rule . . . aren't they?

IBM GLOBAL SURVEY

In October 2008, IBM announced the results of a study of over 1500 change managers from 15 countries. The findings make worrying reading. The study, entitled *Making Change Work* (Somers, NY: IBM Corporation; 2008), reveals that almost 60% of business change projects fail to meet their objectives. In some organisations – the bottom 20% of the sample – project success rates were around 8%. Changing mindsets and attitudes was found to be the biggest challenge to implementing change, followed by corporate culture.

Sadly, the anecdotal evidence that change is often badly handled is backed up by research such as the IBM. We have seen too many change projects begin with high ideals, corporate fanfares and generous funding, only to run into the sand having achieved little more than a relabelling of roles and thicker procedures manuals. Some actually seem to cause more harm than good. But we can't ignore the need for change. Somehow we have to get better at it.

The reason so much change goes wrong is that we seem to forget that any change that matters concerns the way people *think* and *act*. This is inevitable because every organisation is first and foremost a network of people. Even the most hi-tech company relies on people working together to provide products for other people. When we think about change, it is vital to remember that what we are dealing with is not primarily a structure or a process but people in a network of relationships. Although this may seems obvious, it is remarkable how often we seem to miss this point.

In his excellent book *Images of Organisation*,[1] Gareth Morgan points out that we frequently use language from the world of machines to talk about organisations. We talk of them as 'a well-oiled machine' or as 'running like clockwork'. This is indicative of the way some organisations, particularly bureaucracies, are run. Jobs and tasks are standardised and tightly defined. Skills, knowledge and even sometimes values and attitudes are measured against competence frameworks, and adjustments made when the person does not conform to the standard. This tendency to talk about organisations in an impersonal or technical way may reflect a reluctance to acknowledge the often messy reality of managing people. It is as though we would like management to be as simple, straightforward and predictable as operating a machine, so we talk and plan as if this were the case. But this approach does not help in the business of changing hearts and minds; in fact it gets in the way.

This chapter looks at the most common approach to change in organisations and why it doesn't work. In the next chapter we will go on to suggest some approaches more likely to result in changed behaviour and less likely to simply annoy or offend the very people we rely on.

SOCIAL SYSTEMS AT WORK

We've known for some time that treating people like parts of a machine doesn't work. Way back in the 1940s, managers at a coal mine wanted to increase productivity by introducing a shift system, greater specialisation and new technology – the 'longwall method'. On paper it made perfect sense and promised greater efficiency. At the time the miners worked in self-selecting, self-managing teams – the 'shortwall method'. But when the new method was introduced, it failed to bring the hoped-for benefits, mainly because of the disruption it created in the way people worked. The small independent teams were broken up and the knock-on effects included absenteeism and lack of cooperation. The happy ending to the story is that a third method was introduced – the 'composite longwall method' – which gave back some responsibility to the team and reintroduced multi-skilled roles. This third method was more rewarding, both economically and socially, than the longwall method.[2]

THE DIRECTIVE APPROACH: GOOD FOR MACHINES, BAD FOR PEOPLE

Rigid, step-by-step instructions are ideal for operating or fixing machines. A piece of equipment like an electric drill has no ideas to offer, no ability to be inspired or offended, and no aspirations to be anything other than what it was produced to be. When you need to add a sanding attachment or replace a worn-out drill bit the drill feels neither pain nor joy. You don't need to persuade the drill to accept the new part or explain why change is needed. Provided all the pieces are present and correct, all you have to do is implement the instructions. However, this approach is also mistakenly used in organisations and anyone who has worked in a big organisation will have experienced such change. Like machine manuals the instructions come from afar (in this case, top management), they are essentially non-negotiable and they are expected to work in the same standardised way regardless of the people involved. The appeal of this machine-like way of introducing organisational change is obvious. Superficially it is clear, simple and logical. Above all, it appears to be fast. You simply tell people what you want them to do.

Research carried out by Professor Malcolm Higgs[3] labelled this approach as 'directive' and found that it was the most common, but also the least successful, way of bringing change to an organisation. No matter how much we try to bring predictability to organisations, through uniforms, grades, job descriptions and procedures, the directive approach to change will, more often than not, fail. It's not that procedures or standards are wrong. On the contrary, when it comes to assembling equipment, processing an insurance claim or making safety checks they are helpful or even essential. It's just that when we want people to change what they do or how they do it, we have to treat them as *people*, not as parts.

SELF-ASSEMBLY CHANGE

Higgs found that some organisations used what he labelled a 'self-assembly' approach to change. This pushes responsibility for implementation to the local managers and gives them tool kits and templates to implement the change. At first glance this seems more empowering but in reality it leaves very little freedom for local initiative. Like buying self-assembly furniture, you have the freedom to assemble it yourself but there is still only one way to do it. Like directive change, self-assembly change is negatively correlated with success.

For the sake of accuracy, we should point out that there are some circumstances in which the directive approach works very well with people. If you were trapped in a burning building you would want simple and clear instructions from the fire officer. You would not even care whether he said 'please' or 'thank you'. In such a situation you would gladly be told what to do. Why? Because we do not have to be convinced of the need for immediate change, because we know the cost of not changing would be too high and because the fire officer is the undisputed expert in what should be done. The more these factors are present – such as when my car breaks down, or when we need emergency medical help – the more we will tolerate, even welcome, the directive approach.

But in most organisational change these factors are less evident or even completely absent. If a manager announces a change to a familiar and comfortable shift pattern, staff might legitimately ask questions like 'Why should I change?' or 'What was wrong with the old system?' When confronted with these questions, the instinctive response of many managers is to push harder, becoming both more defensive and insistent (as managers we sometimes act like the stereotypical British person abroad, who expects to be understood if they speak their own language both slowly and loudly and whose response to an evident lack of understanding is even more volume!). A manager might win the battle of wills that ensues, but goodwill and credibility are the casualties. It is all too easy to see organisational change as a battle. We quickly label those who oppose our view as 'resistors', forgetting that when we ourselves oppose change that is imposed upon us we tend to see ourselves as the voice of sanity and reason.

THE CHANGE EQUATION: WHY DO PEOPLE SOMETIMES RESIST CHANGE?

A good way to avoid change management becoming needlessly confrontational is to think about why an individual might not willingly go along with the changes we propose. One way of doing this is to use one of the many variations of the Change Equation originated by Richard Beckhard and Wendy Pritchard[4] (attributed to David Gleicher), and later simplified by Kathleen D Dannemillar and Robert Jacobs.[5] This works on the principle that an individual's willingness to change will depend on three factors: D – their dissatisfaction with the status quo, V – their vision of what is possible and F – their knowledge of the practical first steps. This can be expressed as $D \times V \times F > R$, where R is resistance to change. In other words, unless someone is dissatisfied with the way things are, shares the vision of how things could be better and knows what the next steps are, they are likely to resist the change. This helps us avoid applying the blanket term 'resistor' to anyone who does not willingly embrace our change. Some may resist it because they are quite happy with the status quo.

Others may share your desire to see change but not share your particular vision of the future. It could even be that some share your vision and share your dissatisfaction but do not know what to do next. It is sloppy and inaccurate to see all resistors as lazy, stupid or Luddite. In short it is dangerous to assume that all those who are having difficulty accepting the change are doing so for the same reason.

Using the change equation involves seeing things from the individual position of those whose support you hope to enlist.

Why might someone prefer to keep things as they are? Perhaps the proposed change disrupts valued working relationships or maybe they were part of setting up the system you want to change.

If staff don't share your vision, could it be that you didn't involve them in creating the vision, or perhaps they have an even better way forward?

Or is their resistance nothing more than insufficient clarity about what they are expected to do next? In such circumstances it is pointless to keep enthusing about the vision.

Asking such questions enables us to take action likely to reduce resistance.

The change equation reminds us that genuine involvement always makes change more likely to succeed. We say genuine involvement to distinguish it from times when organisations just go through the motions. Such dishonesty contributes to the high levels of cynicism present in many workplaces. We know of one organisation that carefully consults before major decisions – but offers only one option for consultation!

IF DIRECTIVE CHANGE DOESN'T WORK, WHY DO WE KEEP DOING IT?

You now know that the directive approach takes no account of the change equation or of why people respond differently to change. It relies on the power of the organisation's hierarchy to force compliance through discipline or other sanctions, rather than the winning of hearts and minds. If the goal should be change that is willingly embraced, this approach will fail in almost all circumstances. The puzzle is why, when we know the directive approach to be so flawed, do managers so often resort to it? We would suggest three main reasons.

1 **This is the way we've always done it.**

We meet many managers whose approach to change is simply a reflection of how they themselves have been treated. They have been browbeaten or compelled into change and now they, in turn, use similar methods. Even though they may have suffered personally from directive change they readily adopt the same technique. This is rarely a thought-through philosophy but rather an ingrained set of assumptions about how management should be practised – all the more powerful because it is unconscious. In our programmes we often come across these assumptions expressed as if they were unquestionable truths. 'Noone likes change' some managers tell us, or 'You have to show them who is in charge' or even 'People will always try to get away with the minimum'. None of these things are true and such comments often reveal more about the people who say them than their staff. Even where managers can see that the directive approach is counter productive it is easy to conclude that there is no alternative. Corporate culture, reality TV programmes and popular stereotypes all reinforce the idea that 'hire 'em, fire 'em' macho management is the way it should be done. Even many management books promote an approach to change that is little more than a polite version of command and control, directive change.

2   **We'd love to involve staff more but we just don't have the time.**
    Involving staff, genuinely listening to their concerns, being ready to incorporate other people's ideas – these things take time, effort and character. So it is tempting to resort to directive change, particularly if that is how you yourself are being managed. But the consequence of trying to save time by just telling people what to do is that we will spend even more time further down the line either unpicking our mistakes or struggling against the additional 'drag' that diminished goodwill creates. Carefully involving and listening to your team in change is like digging the foundations of a house. To the uneducated it seems like you are not making much progress – no walls have been erected – but without it changes may well be unstable and short lived.

3   **Anyone can see that this is what we must do!**
    This mistake comes from assuming that you see the world the way I do. It is what happens when we think something is so obviously the right thing to do that we assume everyone else must agree. We start in a new job and immediately see several things we can easily improve. It doesn't occur to us to even see this as change, it is just improvement or updating, and so we simply announce what will happen. The resistance and resentment then take us by surprise. 'What is wrong with these people' we say, and rather than see any problem with what we have done, we quickly label those who have questioned our action as resistors or troublemakers. This can also be seen when groups of managers work together on strategy. For months they study the situation and consider the options until the way forward seems self evidently clear. Clear, that is, to them. To the rest of the staff, who have not had weeks or months to go though the same thought processes, it is often a new and unproved solution to a problem they didn't know they had.

    As we think about how change is typically done in organisations, it is clear that directive, top-down, machine-style change is the wrong approach in almost every single situation. But it is also clear that doing it this way is an easy trap to fall into. Perhaps the biggest problem is that many managers don't really see, or even look for, a viable alternative. All around we see this style of managing being practised and preached. For some, their confrontational style is a badge of honour. They seem to relish having a reputation for being aggressive – mistaking this for directness; or for being cynical – mistaking this for wisdom. Such role models abound in management, politics and the professions. The result of this is that organisations are constantly trying to fix the problems which were caused by their last solution.

Leading people through change is far more than a technical exercise. It requires courage and care as well as an analytical mind. One good definition of leadership is that the leader brings hope. Sadly we often see people being pushed into change by force rather than pulled through it by a compelling vision of how things will be better.

The good news is that there is an alternative to directive-change management. But it requires us to think in a different way about our teams and organisations, a more holistic way. It also means that we may have to go against the flow and work more thoughtfully. The next chapter explains more about this different way of leading change.

Before you read on, think about the most recent changes you have introduced.
➤ How much involvement did your team have in shaping the changes?
➤ If some people opposed the changes, how did you deal with them?

REFERENCES

1 Morgan G. *Images of Organisation*. Thousand Oaks: Sage; 1998.
2 Trist EL, Higgin GW, Murray H, *et al. Organisational Choice*. London: Tavistock; 1963.
3 Higgs MJ, Rowland D. *Change and its Leadership: is it time for a change in our thinking?* ECLO Conference. Prague; 2006. (Paper received Academic Award of Merit Distinction.)
4 Beckhard R, Pritchard W. *Changing the Essence: the art of creating and leading fundamental change in organizations*. San Francisco: Jossey-Bass; 1992.
5 Dannemiller KD, Jacobs RW. Changing the way organizations change: a revolution of common sense. *J Appl Behav Sci*. 1992; **28**(4): 480–98.

CHAPTER 4

Tools for change

We hope that the last chapter has made you think about the need to do change differently. What underlies the *unsuccessful* approaches is seeing organisations and teams only as machines and seeing people only as parts. This leads to a style of change management that, at very best, brings short-term results. Instead, we need to remind ourselves that a team is a network of human relationships and that we manage people, not components. Without this awareness we will miss many of the factors that influence change. We have to remember that we employ whole people, with emotions and ambitions as well as skills and knowledge. To manage change successfully we have to think about wholes as well as parts.

THINKING IN WHOLES PART 1: THE ICEBERG

Imagine an iceberg.[1] The part of it that is above the water can be many metres high. But there is another part below the waterline. In fact, around seven-eighths of the iceberg is out of sight under the waves. Because this part is hidden it is especially dangerous to passing ships.

Now think about your team or organisation. There are many things about it that are either obvious or easy to find out. These include structures, products or services, the number of staff and their jobs and qualifications, plans and strategies, performance targets . . . the list goes on. This kind of information is set down in words and numbers and is accessible to managers. Like the tip of the iceberg these things are easy to see, but we shouldn't make the mistake of thinking that they are all there is. There are other factors, less easily available and usually not written down: about morale, about how people get on with each other and how they have been treated in the past, their hopes and fears, the organisational culture, levels of trust, attitudes to customers, etc. These are insubstantial, hard to define things that nevertheless have a huge impact on how the organisation behaves. When it comes to managing change this information is just as important as the written-down stuff, but it is hidden, as it were, below the waterline.

Above the waterline	Below the waterline
The formal management structure	Who really has the power
Skills profile	Personality profile
Checks and audits	Trust and mistrust
Investment in new developments	Creativity and initiative
Strategy	What we really think will happen
Formal communication	Informal networks
Staff – numbers, qualifications, grades	Staff – motivation, hopes and fears
Information	Intuition
Procedures – what we do	Culture – how we do it
Logic	Wisdom
Financial history	Staff memory

We're certainly not saying ignore the things above the waterline. Structures, budgets, procedures and the like are all very important. But the tendency of organisations is to act is if that is all there is. This is so ingrained that when we talk about organisational change, one of the first things many managers do is to start fiddling with the organisational chart.

It is interesting that when we begin consulting to an organisation, one of the first things they usually provide for us is the wiring diagram (again a machine metaphor). It contains the job titles and reporting arrangements together with handwritten amendments that signify that there are vacancies or that someone's responsibilities have been changed recently. Information on what it is like to work there, how people are coping, where the ideas come from and who really pulls the strings cannot be gleaned from such two-dimensional data and may take some time to unearth.

But even if we have taken care of all the structures, numbers, policies and strategies the task is still incomplete. It's worth remembering that with goodwill and enthusiasm almost any structure or process can be made to work, whereas without them the best new strategic initiative will fail.

Whole people

These below-the-waterline issues are a reminder that organisations employ whole people. Along with their work-related skills come all their other human attributes, and we ignore them at our peril. An example of this is 'survivor syndrome' where those who keep their jobs at a time when many of their colleagues have been made redundant experience fear, anger and distrust. At first glance this seems paradoxical; we might think that such people would feel only relief and gratitude that they had survived the cuts. But this fails to take into account the complexities of human behaviour. Such survivors may feel guilty, resentful on behalf of colleagues who lost their jobs, or hard done by because they must now work harder to cover jobs that have been axed. They often feel less able to trust their managers, are more apprehensive about the future and less likely to take initiative, lest they are next for the chop.

A study by Kusum Sander and Susan Vinnicrombe, Cranfield School of Management,[2] found that managers who lead such 'downsizing' exercises were often 'over-optimistic and in some instances over-simplistic'. They grossly underestimated the human impact of job cuts. Instead of simply reducing labour costs they found that they had set other forces in motion that led to a less motivated, less innovative and more stressed workforce. This simplistic optimism is the result of seeing only the tip of the iceberg. Above-the-waterline thinking only sees the numbers and the costs. But below the waterline lie forces that mean that the impact of such changes can reverberate around the organisation for many years, sapping morale and tainting communication between staff and management. The managers in the study had not thought about wholes, they had treated people as if they were simply concerned with having a job and earning money. If this were the case, 'survivor syndrome' would not exist. But real, whole people are also concerned about colleagues, about loyalty, about fairness. They care about whether management can be trusted.

To remember that we manage whole people is not simply a matter of ethics. It is not something we should bear in mind just when we have the luxury of time and resources. *It is the basis of good management.*

Another common example is when we merge teams or organisations. The following story is a combination of several similar case studies.

A few years ago a large international company decided to buy a much smaller company who specialised in software design. On paper (above the waterline), it looked perfect. The bigger company needed the innovative designs of the smaller one, which in turn needed the financial resources and international networks of the larger organisation. Everything was done carefully and with due diligence. The lawyers and accountants did their job thoroughly.

However, it soon became obvious that all was not well. One of the principal reasons was that the staff of the software design company were now working in a very different culture. Instead of being part of a flexible small team with a flat structure and lots of autonomy, they were now a very small part of a very large corporation. Their flexibility was constrained by corporate controls they could not influence; they even found that they could not simply buy the computer hardware they wanted because it exceeded the standard corporate specification. They no longer felt like a self-determining, close-knit team on an adventure, they felt like cogs in the corporate machine. Discontent grew and performance began to tail off.

All the reasons for this setback came from below the waterline. The impact of the takeover on the ethos and culture of the smaller company was ignored. It was assumed that its staff would simply continue doing the same sort of work. Above-the-waterline factors had been beautifully managed, below-the-waterline issues had been ignored or discounted.

A participant on a Vital Signs programme told us of how his team was asked to merge with another team as part of a wider reorganisation. Both teams were effective and respect was mutual. Also, the reasoning behind the merger was accepted by all. Everything looked good on paper; a logical combination of two good teams to create an even bigger, better one. The problems only began to emerge when the teams began meeting together. What had been missed was that although both teams were effective, they were effective in very different ways. One team had noisy, lively meetings and a loose structure held together by longstanding relationships between team members. The other team was much more hierarchical and paid closer attention to procedure and protocol. These cultures did not mix well. Tensions became apparent and would have adversely affected performance had there not been some wise leadership and a readiness to compromise. Again, the factors that threatened success were located below the waterline and were to do with the very different cultures and histories of each team. We must recognise that these sorts of issues are every bit as deserving of management attention as structures and finances.

Involving people

As a conscientious manager you might now be asking how you can possibly take account of all the below-the-waterline factors in your team. How can you be aware of the complexities of personalities, history and relationships that can exist even in a small team? The answer of course is that you cannot, but your people can. This is why it is critical to involve people in the change process.

Even the best manager cannot take account of everything that is going on below the waterline in their team. But if staff are allowed to shape or even drive the change themselves, we don't have to! The more change is imposed from above, the more below the waterline problems it will stir up, in turn requiring more management time to deal with those (avoidable) problems. To be effective, involvement must be genuine. In other words, we must give staff time and opportunity to influence our decisions. Even better, we should delegate to staff the authority to constantly improve the way they work. We can help them to do this by training them in one of the many improvement processes that have been tested and tried in organisational settings. But once they have the skills and the information they need, we should get out of their way! We are both constantly inspired by the vision and courage of managers who do this. On a large scale there is the example of Ricardo Semler who revolutionised his company by allowing staff to set their own wage rises and appoint their own bosses (Semler's book, *Maverick*, is on our Vital Signs recommended reading list). On a smaller scale we have found team leaders willing to trust their staff to set rotas and bring in changes of their own.

Time and again we see that almost all staff, given the opportunity and the training, will innovate, experiment and act responsibly. Whether you will allow them to do this depends, to a large extent, on your beliefs about people.

ASSUMPTIONS ABOUT STAFF – WHAT DO YOU THINK?

Think of the way staff are managed in your organisation. What assumptions underpin the way we treat them? Whatever our website or annual report might say, our day-to-day practices and procedures tell the real story. Constant checks, controls, audits and rigid procedures tell staff that we assume they are untrustworthy and unable to make good decisions. These sorts of assumptions annoy Tom Peters,[3] the influential management writer: 'people in enterprise . . . in government are by and large well intentioned. They'd like to get things done. To be of service to others. But they're thwarted at every step of the way by absurd organisational barriers and by the egos of petty tyrants . . .'

Do you agree?

Allow us to ask you a few searching questions.
- ➤ Would you deliberately defraud your employers?
- ➤ Do you always do the minimum amount of work you can get away with?
- ➤ Do you only ever do good work if someone is checking up on you?

Of course not! You would probably be offended if a colleague or boss asked you these questions, and rightly so. But if this is the case, why are we content to devise and implement systems that seem to be founded on the assumption that our staff are either stupid or untrustworthy? Perhaps we think that honesty and responsibility can only be found within those in, or on their way to, the boardroom. Of course we accept that there are a small number of staff who may take advantage of freedoms given to them. But is that a good enough reason to stifle the imagination and initiative of all of their colleagues?

THINKING IN WHOLES PART 2: COMPLEX SYSTEMS

So far, we have argued that we need to see our staff as whole people, not just packages of skills, knowledge or muscle. But we need to go a step further in this holistic thinking. We need to stand back for a minute and look at our team in its context. This next section invites you to think differently about your team and its network of relationships with the wider organisation – the whole system.

Earlier in the chapter we talked about how managers often talk and think about organisations as if they were machines, and how this leads us to ignore or minimise people issues. But machine thinking has another drawback: it leads us to take the wrong approach to change and problem solving. Let us explain. Machines are often complicated, so if a machine needs repair we need to try to isolate the fault from amongst many possible causes. Using a process of elimination we keep breaking the machine down to smaller and smaller parts till the faulty part is identified. We can then replace the part and the machine will work again. This process of *scaling down* is useful in highlighting the exact location of the problem.

Complex versus complicated

One of us recently took a very expensive valve-powered guitar amplifier to a shop to be repaired. The technician quickly established that the valves were fine, the speaker was working and the controls were all functional. He successfully isolated the problem as being in the connection between the speaker and amplifier. He scaled down and successfully fixed the amplifier. Once the problem was identified he didn't have to think of the whole amplifier, just the part that had a problem. Valve amplifiers are complicated. There are lots of wires, circuits and knobs and it takes time and experience to know where everything is and what it does. But it can be known. Once we have learned how it is all connected, it won't change. Provided all parts are working we can predict its performance exactly. So even when something is complicated, it can, with skill, be managed or predicted.

However, when I take my valve amplifier to a jam session with other musicians and we improvise together, even if you knew lots about us and our music, you could not know in advance what we would play. There are simply too many variables to be known. Even the musicians themselves could not predict how the improvised piece will turn out, and they are the ones playing it! This is the difference between complicated and complex problems. Complicated problems may take a long time to understand fully, but they can be understood and therefore controlled. Complex problems, on the other hand, can never be fully understood and therefore cannot be controlled, they can only be influenced. Sending a rocket to Mars is complicated. Bringing up a child is complex.

MANAGEMENT AND ALL THAT JAZZ

Managing a team or an organisation is a complex task. Several management writers have used the image of a musical jam to express this.[4] *See*, for example F Barrett. (1998). They argue that because of the number of variables and factors beyond their control, a good management team is like a jazz band. They might know the key and roughly what the structure of the piece should be, but they have to constantly change and adapt according to what happens around them. If you watch musicians improvising, they are listening carefully to each other, sometimes they stop playing altogether, and sometimes they take a lead. They often seem to 'just know' when the rhythm or feel of the music needs to change. This seems to us like a good way of understanding management in the real world. It is not so much about predicting and controlling, but more about listening, adapting and seizing opportunity. In musical terms, it's more like a jazz band improvising than an orchestra playing a written-down score. Top-down, highly controlled change in such circumstances is just inappropriate.

When we treat complex problems as it they were merely complicated, we end up in trouble. Using chemical fertilisers to increase crop yield is a good example of this. If we scale down, all we see is the need to grow more and grow it faster. Chemical fertilisers enable us to do this, therefore problem solved! But if we scale up, we see that crops and fields are part of a larger ecosystem and that the chemicals in the fertiliser are washed into the rivers and have unpredictable effects on other plants and animals. Ultimately the action we took to increase land fertility inhibits fertility in other parts of the ecosystem because of pollution. An ecosystem is more than complicated, it is complex. If we try to use the same approach as we use for machines – scaling down – we may do serious damage.

Now instead of an ecosystem, think of a family with a poorly behaved child. A moment's thought will tell us that although it is the child who is misbehaving, if we want to understand what is going on we need to look at not just the child but also the wider family situation. Instead of *scaling down*, we need to *scale up*. If we simply look at the child we may end up blaming them for things beyond their control, such as poor parenting or bullying. A child's behaviour is a complex issue that cannot be treated like a machine problem.

Similarly it can be dangerous to use a machine approach with a team. For instance, imagine a team which normally performs well but where one member's attendance and performance start to decline. Scaling down would lead us to focus on that one person and their particular issues. We may even use a competence framework to assess their performance and send them for corrective training. If this fails to solve the problem, disciplinary action is the next option. But wait a minute.

Team performance is complex and is about more than the individual members. It is also about the relationships *between* the members. If one member is being bullied or undermined by another, the first signs may be a drop in the performance of the person being intimidated. In this case, homing in on this person will not solve the problem. Instead of breaking the situation down into smaller and smaller parts, we need to step back and look at it in its entirety. To understand performance issues in a team member, we have to look at the whole team, we have to *scale up*.

Teams and families share certain attributes.

➤ The relationships between the different people are crucial in determining what happens.

➤ They can be influenced but not controlled or predicted in detail.

➤ Changes to one person will affect all the others.

A term that can be applied to teams, families and ecosystems is *complex systems*. Other examples of complex systems are financial markets and the human body. They have a number of interconnected parts or elements which share the same environment but which each have some ability to act autonomously.

Lessons from working with complex systems

Much has been written about complex systems. If you want to pursue the subject in more depth we would strongly recommend *The Fifth Discipline* by Peter Senge.[5] But there are some profound lessons to be drawn from *systems thinking*, as it is known, that all managers need to consider:

➤ a few simple rules are better than many

➤ manage thoughtfully

➤ all change starts with me.

A few simple rules

Complex systems cannot be successfully controlled. If you try to control them the consequences may be both negative and unpredictable. Despite this, organisations are full of the language of control. Plans, procedures and job descriptions all give the impression that things are under control. You may even think of your team in this way, considering it to be a resource that can be controlled and utilised to complete various tasks. But we should never forget that organisations are made up of people who, as people, can make choices about where they work and the level of commitment they bring to work.

Control in organisations is expressed in structures and procedures designed to guide behaviour by limiting choice. This is usually done for good reasons, such as accident prevention or speeding up decision-making. But an excess of rules and regulations will lead to a reduction in the ability of people in the organisation to use their critical faculties to innovate, to take initiative – to make decisions for themselves. We see this in the experiences of long-term prisoners who are released back into society, people who leave the armed forces or the citizens of countries where communist regimes have been supplanted by emerging democracies. Having lived for so long in an environment where so many decisions are made on their behalf, a disturbingly large number of them find it hard to cope in so-called normal society. Having been used to a very limited amount of control over their own lives, the self-determination and resilience needed to cope in a world full of uncertainty and choice is a real challenge, at least in the short term.

While prison and the armed forces may be extreme examples of controlled environments, many organisations have similar approaches to proceduralising their work and limiting the scope for individual choice. In most public service organisations the tasks undertaken by staff are partly or completely governed by procedure. Each procedure exists for good reasons, they are intended to eliminate waste, reduce accidents, prevent discrimination and a wealth of other laudable objectives. But the cumulative effect is to sap initiative and creativity. Even worse, they can unwittingly create a perception amongst staff that they are not to be trusted, and that if there were no rules liberties would be taken, dishonesty would be the norm and backsliding would be commonplace.

Sometimes the same organisations that impose these controls then attempt to encourage the innovative behaviour which they have unintentionally suppressed. One of us witnessed a public sector CEO exhorting his senior staff to be creative in their planning. He encouraged them to think outside the box and to take risks. He demanded that they be radical and questioning. After this rousing speech, his deputy took the stage and told the managers exactly how they should submit their plans. He specified the template they should adhere to, and the font style and size they must use. He laid down the exact process they should follow and the deadline for each stage. The contradiction between the two messages was painfully obvious but not up for discussion. 'We want you to innovate', the organisation seemed to be saying 'but you must do it in exactly this way'.

WHEN SAFETY CONTROLS REDUCE SAFETY

Road safety has been a big concern for policymakers for some time. As more and more cars come onto our roads we have tried to reduce risk through ever-increasing control. Speed limits, warning signs and traffic lights have been seen as the way to avoid accidents. However, in the town of Drachten in Holland accidents have been dramatically reduced by doing just the opposite. Removing the traffic lights at one major junction led to accidents falling from 36 in the previous four years to just 2 in two years. Interestingly, traffic flow through the junction increased. Such 'shared space' projects have deliberately blurred the boundaries between road and kerb and encouraged pedestrians, cyclists and drivers to be more aware of each other.[6] The result is more careful behaviour as people realise they must take responsibility for their own actions. Early experiments in the UK, such as removing railings along a stretch of a high street in London, have also been encouraging. Conventional wisdom was that accidents could be reduced by controlling where people crossed the road. This appears not to be true as pedestrian casualties in the area decreased three times faster than the London average when road users were handed back their 'freedom'.

So what's going on here? It seems that our instinctive response to accidents, i.e. to increase controls and regulation, may actually be counter productive. Perhaps the more I feel my behaviour is externally regulated by traffic lights, barriers and pedestrian crossings, the less I will think about how I'm driving. So action taken to reduce accidents can sometimes have exactly the opposite effect. Brake, the UK road-safety charity, while reminding us that we cannot assume it would work in all situations, recognises that reducing road markings and road signs has reduced accidents in several towns. (See www.brake.org.uk.)

Like overprotective parents who, in shielding their children from risk, produce children unable to manage risk themselves, managers who try to make their staff act in certain ways often get the opposite of what they say they want. This seems paradoxical, but systems-thinking helps us understand what is happening. In imposing too many controls and procedures, we are actually training our staff to take less and less responsibility for their own actions. However, faced with the failure of controls to achieve compliance, the usual response is not to question the need for control but . . . you guessed it . . . to impose yet more controls. Hans Monderman, the initiator of the road safety experiments referred to in the box above, made a comment that many managers would do well to note: *'when faced with a safety problem, most engineers tend to install something additional. My instinct is always to take something away.'*[7]

So, if too much control can create the very problems we are trying to solve, what can be done? The answer is not a comforting one for those managers who find it hard to trust their staff. Controls need to be kept to a minimum – a few simple non-negotiables – and staff need to be encouraged to use their own judgement. For this to work, it is essential that performance issues are addressed promptly and clearly because, if we are relying on trust rather than control, when trust breaks down it must be swiftly remedied. Involving people does not mean abdicating management responsibility.

Professor Malcolm Higgs, who has highlighted the ineffectiveness of directive change[8] (*see* Chapter 3) has described an approach that is much more likely to succeed. He calls this 'emergent' change, and it is characterised by a few big rules and loosely set direction. Changes can be initiated anywhere in the organisation, particularly at the 'business end', where staff are in direct contact with clients or customers. Instead of templates or top-down directives, there is an emphasis on innovation and improvisation.

TRUSTING STAFF TO SORT IT OUT

The benefits of giving staff a few simple non-negotiables and then letting them get on with it are illustrated in the very mundane issue of managing rotas and leave requests. In one example we came across, a health manager had tried to avoid having too few staff on duty on clinic days by imposing a requirement for staff to give 6 weeks notice of any days they wanted to take as holiday. The result? Prevented from taking annual leave when they sometimes genuinely needed it at short notice, staff who needed time off would take sick leave. To make things worse, they would not just be absent the day of the clinic as this would be too obvious. Instead they would take another day or two. The control not only failed to achieve its objective, it actually increased absence as staff were forced to subvert the system in order to cope with eventualities such as breakdowns in childcare.

In contrast, we met a wise nurse manager who had addressed a similar issue by giving staff a few non-negotiables such as the levels of cover needed and allowing them to work out their own system. The staff devised their own principles, such as giving preference for holidays out of term time to those with school-age children, and sorted themselves out. The resultant peer-to-peer obligations were much more effective at producing sustainable changed behaviour than any management manual or policy.

We are not suggesting anarchy. There must always be limits to what can be done and what the organisation will allow. But if these are kept to a minimum, the considerable potential of your staff to make good decisions and improve the way they work is more likely to be released. Rosabeth Moss Kanter, in her book *The Change Masters*,[9] argues that whilst power can corrupt, so can powerlessness! In other words, take power away and smart people will find a way round the system (remember the sick leave example above). Technically it is corrupt, or at best, devious, but managers need to remember that it is a response to a perceived lack of trust, not a reason to trust even less!

Manage thoughtfully

> *The brain is a wonderful organ. It starts working the moment you get up in the morning and does not stop until you get into the office.*
>
> Robert Frost

Management is plagued by the need to be seen to take action. Pressure from senior management, shareholders or government ministers lead managers to do things which are designed as much to show that something is being done as to solve the problem. Unfortunately though, ill-considered action can actually make things worse.

Once, after a coaching session, a health manager said to one of us that he'd found it all very helpful and that he was now going to the hospital library to write down his reflections. When asked why he wasn't going back to his office he said 'that wouldn't work, they've installed motion-triggered lights to save energy. If I sit still for any length of time, the lights go off'. While we applaud every effort to save energy, installing motion-triggered lights in a manager's office sends a strong message about what was expected of that manager. 'Don't spend time thinking,' is the implicit message, 'move about, look busy – do things'.

One manager told me that she would love to be able to manage more thoughtfully but the never-ending stream of staff who came into her office seeking assistance meant that she had no time. I asked what she did when they asked for help. 'I help them,' she said, 'I solve their problems'. She bemoaned the fact that her staff seemed unable to deal with issues themselves. But as we talked further she began to see how her 'leave it with me' approach encouraged her staff to keep bringing their problems to her. She was, in effect, training them to be dependent. She had created the very problem she complained of by rewarding staff for *not* taking initiative. Only when she stepped back from the situation was she able to see the repetitive loop of behaviour she had established with her staff.

Another manager with a similar issue described what happened when she decided to break this loop. As a smart, no-nonsense manager she had revelled in her ability to solve problems for her staff. After attending Vital Signs she changed her approach. She told how a particular member of staff who frequently asked for help came into her office with a problem. But instead of telling her what to do or saying 'Leave it with me', the manager asked a series of open questions to help her team member decide what to do for herself. Even more importantly, she listened carefully to the responses. 'It was like a truth serum!', the manager reflected. The member of staff left her office having not only answered her own question, but also having gained some valuable insight into her own behaviour.

Active listening: the importance of shutting up!

If we are honest, much of our 'listening' is simply waiting for a chance to get our point across. In our programmes we often ask managers to practise what is often called active listening. This involves listening carefully in order to genuinely understand. Instead of leaping to conclusions or suggesting ways to fix the problem before it is understood, the active listener asks open questions and helps the other person clarify their thinking by talking it through. Managers are always surprised by how hard this is to do and even more surprised by the number of times it leads to new insights and solutions on both sides.

In one organisation we worked with, headquarters staff grew frustrated with what they saw as the failure of regional staff to correctly fill in the forms that provided them with performance information. So they took action and made the form longer and more detailed. To their annoyance, the new forms were completed even more sketchily than the old ones. Their action had failed and they were convinced that the blame lay with regional staff. From the perspective of the staff in the regions, however, the old forms were an exercise in pointlessness. They did not receive any useful feedback from them and were unsure as to why they had to be completed. So when the new, even longer forms appeared, their puzzlement turned to quiet rebellion and they were even less inclined to provide the information.

Action had been taken. No one could accuse the headquarters staff of complacency. But because it was not thought through it just made things worse. Headquarters failed to see the complex system they were part of, and they could not see the connections between their actions and the behaviour they complained about.

In all these cases, the actions of the managers had created the very problems they were now struggling with. But until they stood back and saw what was going on they were unable to discern this. As far as they were concerned the problem lay with their staff and their inability to make good decisions. But before we get too critical of these managers, remember that this is an easy trap to fall into. Unthinkingly, we all do things that satisfy our need to do something quickly but which result in other problems further down the line. Think about it. It is likely that several of the things you have had to sort out today are the direct result of previous actions you have taken. Peter Senge calls this 'the illusion of taking charge,'[5] where we act in a way we feel is decisive but without sufficient thought for the consequences. But because organisations and teams are complex systems, where all the parts are connected, there will always be a consequence. However, unless we take the time to stand back and look at what is going on in the whole system (i.e. scale up) we may never see the connections between yesterday's decisions and today's problems.

To manage well, you must manage thoughtfully. And to do this takes time, space and a different way of thinking about the context you manage. Stepping back from the urgency of everyday demands is not always easy. So here are some practical ways to allow yourself to manage more thoughtfully.

➤ **Time out.** Take your immediate team away from the office, ward or department for at least a couple of hours. Do it every 6 months even if you are feeling snowed under. The busier you are, the more you need to step back. Don't have a formal agenda – this will mean you'll just think about issues in the same old ways. Instead, use a process like the one we describe later in this chapter (*see* 'Vision of the future', p.68). The aim is to think in a different way than you normally do, so don't have a normal meeting. Sometimes we ask teams to draw a picture of how they want things to be, or of how relationships with other departments are. We have often found that teams surprise themselves with the insights they gain from the *process* of drawing as well as from the finished picture. Make sure you end the session by agreeing some conclusions and actions to turn your insights into improvements. Also, if you are the manager, don't fall in to the trap of feeling you are the one who must have the best ideas or suggestions. Bearing in mind Belbin's team roles from Chapter 2, you need to make room for the gifts of other people. Your job is just to make sure the best ideas are not lost.

➤ **Find your balance.** Excuse us for asking, but how is your life going? Do you know what is important to you and where your work fits into this? Are you making time for interests and people outside of work? Thoughtful management is part of a life lived thoughtfully and with a sense of perspective. If you never really have time to sort all this out we recommend you set aside time to do just this. Try reading *Synchronicity* by Joseph Jaworski (San Francisco: Berrett-Koehler; 1996) or book yourself in for a retreat. We recommend Ffald y Brenin (www.ffald-y-brenin.org) in Pembrokeshire, Glenfall House (www. glenfallhouse.org) near Cheltenham or Ampleforth Abbey (www.ampleforth. org.uk) near York. Revisit the personal-development planning section of Chapter 2 and remind yourself that you are a whole person and that your life goals and work objectives cannot be completely disentangled. If thinking about your career and your development provoked some uncomfortable realisations, what could you do about this? We have been inspired by people who have made bold decisions to bring their work into line with their values and principles. One lady we know decided, at the age of 50, to leave her job to start a charity to help the homeless people she saw on her way to work. A nurse manager we worked with made the brave decision to move back to clinical work having realised that hands-on nursing was what she loved. Taking time to be thoughtful helped her reconnect with what, for her, was most important.

➤ **Sort out your diary and desk!** Take control of how you spend your time and the space you work in. Write in time for reading and thinking. Cut out useless meetings. Throw away the journals and papers you are never going to read. If you are regularly taking work home with you, you need to carefully review your priorities. Make your diary work for you, and don't let it become just a record of other peoples' demands on your time!

All change starts with me

If we think of our team as a complex system, more like a living organism than a machine, then we also must accept that we are part of that system and that our attitudes and actions contribute to how the system works. As in the stories of the managers who by solving their staff's problems effectively prevented them from developing problem-solving skills, we are inextricably part of the reasons our team performs well or badly. Therefore I must be part of any change that I implement.

This is the critical difference between machine thinking and systems thinking. If I see my team as a machine that I operate, I can tinker with it, upgrade it and repair it without changing myself. I will tend to impose directive change to control behaviour. While most managers would shrink from using this sort of language, this approach is common – where the manager sees themselves as in some way separate from the team, objectively trying to improve its performance. Systems thinking reminds me that I am part of the team, even if I have a different grade or job title.

Therefore the wise manager first of all considers their own performance.

Albert Schweitzer, musician, philosopher, physician and Nobel Peace Prize winner, said: *'Example is not the main thing in influencing others. It is the only thing.'*

This is, admittedly, more demanding than simply slapping on more performance targets. It also rules out the use of blame as a way of avoiding learning. Often when we discuss these issues with managers on our programmes, they begin to talk about top management, or if we are talking to top management, they talk about the board. 'My boss should be on this programme' they will say, as they use their new insights to critique the performance of the tier above. But this misses the point. The first question for anyone who wants to be a good manager is always *'What can I do differently?'*, because real learning is always expressed in action. Finding other people to blame for our problems is seductive but useless. Seductive because there may well be truth in our accusations, useless because it helps us avoid our part in whatever the problem is. Instead of grappling with the need to raise our own game, our energy goes into trench warfare with the person or department we are blaming. Just as you cannot breathe in and out at the same time, you cannot blame and learn at the same time.

If I want my team to be more flexible and ready to change the way they work, I must first of all apply the question to myself. How open and flexible am I? Am I genuinely ready to hear and take on board corrective feedback? Or do I always somehow find reasons to justify my way of managing? If I want my team to innovate and challenge established practice, how do I react when my way of doing things is challenged?

One of the most profound statements about leading change was made 2000 years ago: *'How can you say to your brother, "Let me take the speck out of your eye", when all the time there is a plank in your own eye?'* [10]

The good manager leads primarily by example, constantly embracing learning and change.

HOW TO ENCOURAGE STAFF ENGAGEMENT

So far we have looked at the bigger picture – the systems of which you and your team are part. We have shown that piecemeal, top-down change not only doesn't tend to work, it actually creates an environment where future success is even less likely. Throughout the last two chapters we have returned to the twin themes of trust and involvement. Here is a practical tool you can use with your staff which combines those two values. It works best when you hold a workshop, time out or away day with your team to consider how your service could change and develop in the future. If a full workshop is too much of a luxury, try it at an extended team meeting.

VISION OF THE FUTURE

If you study management theory books you will probably come across this model:

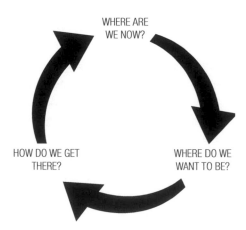

FIGURE 4.1 Planning model I

It is a classic planning model and starts by encouraging people to identify the current position of their team/service/company, etc. Typically this *'Where are we now?'* question is accompanied by a plethora of mapping and measuring exercises, with the result that the team generates activity and performance data, location maps, skill mix tables, financial reports and so on, in order to help them move onto the next question.

'Where do we want to be?' is an attempt to look to the future and identify what changes need to be made. The model concludes with *'How do we get there?'*, leading to the rational and vitally important process of action planning, so that key tasks and responsibilities are clearly laid out.

Having used this model for many years our experiences are mixed. There is no doubt that it is a sensible, logical, clear way of making sense of an otherwise complex set of issues, and yet the changes it stimulates never really seem to 'stir the soul'. We have reflected on what this model actually produces when a group or team uses it, and here are our combined observations on each question.

➤ *Where are we now?* When we work with groups, perhaps on a time out or extended team meeting, we find that (despite us encouraging a balanced approach) this question produces a constant stream of negativity, problems, inadequacies, crises and general despondency. Within a short time, any flip charts or white boards are full of this stuff, regardless of its bearing on the specific issue. It seems that, although the meeting is an attempt to improve things, we focus on how bad they are! The result is that many groups have felt deflated and overwhelmed, before even getting to thinking about the future.

➤ *Where do we want to be?* We find two problems with this question. The first is that the legacy of despondency from the first question tends to stifle creativity and hope. This results in somewhat unambitious ideas for the future, normally based on a few procedural tweaks, and a general sense of 'we will be lucky to turn this round'. The second is that there is no precision in the question. Where is 'Where'? Is it to do with activity, location, results, relationships? Also it tends to rekindle the somewhat sterile debate about the difference between wants and needs. In short its apparent simplicity is its downfall. The discussion it generates is often unfocused and leaves a group no further forward on the essence of the change they are considering.

➤ *How do we get there?* At face value there is nothing wrong with this question. However, it suffers from a lack of clarity and commitment to the other questions. This means that, after a considerable amount of activity mapping and research (question one), a rather restrained and process-based set of ideas for change (question two), the action planning is uninspiring. Trying to get busy staff to take on responsibility for individual actions in the plan is difficult given that there is little to motivate and excite.

Take heart, dear reader. There is an alternative. It takes the same basic enquiry of the original model but injects pace and passion into the process!

Our revised model looks like this:

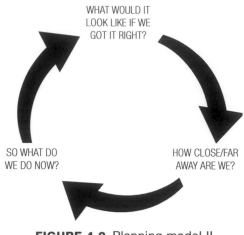

WHAT WOULD IT
LOOK LIKE IF WE
GOT IT RIGHT?

SO WHAT DO
WE DO NOW?

HOW CLOSE/FAR
AWAY ARE WE?

FIGURE 4.2 Planning model II

At first glance it just looks like some minor semantic changes have been made to the original – the sorts of changes that management consultants sometimes get accused of doing and then charging lots of money for!

However, there are profound differences between the two, differences that echo the trust and involvement themes we mentioned earlier. By using the revised model in real-life discussions with staff, remarkable changes take place.

➤ *What would it look like if we got it right?* This question genuinely taps into the staff's motivation to do a good job. It starts on a positive (unlike the *'Where are we now?* question earlier), and allows a whole bunch of 'below-the-waterline' issues to emerge (*see* earlier in this chaper). Teams who have used this model report that the resultant 'vision of the future' contains not only hard activity and performance criteria, but also relationship, feelings atmosphere, impressions, feedback, etc. One team used this question to devise a day in the life of one of their patients in the new care facility being planned, if everything was working as it should. This storyboard contained far more to excite and motivate staff than would have been the case with a classic 'business plan' and, most importantly of all, it was the work of the staff themselves. They were trusted to come up with something that was challenging but doable. Despite management fears, they did not ask for the moon, unrealistic injections of cash and staff, complete freedom to improvise or any other self-indulgent act. They simply thought sensibly about what could be, given the realities they faced – because they were trusted!

➤ *How close/far away are we?* This questions benefits first from the fact that it will be working with a positive vision of the future. Second, semantically it provides balance as it allows a group to identify where things are already going in the desired direction (close), so that those aspects of the work can be celebrated and protected. Also the discussion produced by this question tends to be more upbeat and realistic, even when identifying the issues where there is still much to do (far away). This is partly because those issues are being raised in context and partly because the team already knows it can make things work. Rarely is there the same sense of doom and fatalism associated with the original 'classic' planning model.

➤ *So what do we do now?* This is similar to the third question in the original model but the focus is on getting started now. Some of the actions may take longer to come to fruition so there needs to be some proper sequencing, but the question provokes a real sense of momentum for the team, especially as the response to the earlier questions will have been so positive and useful. Typically we encourage teams to divide their actions into three categories but you may wish to develop your own.

— **Category 1**: Actions that we can take *now*, without further analysis or permission from others.

— **Category 2**: Actions that require more thought and/or approval from beyond the team, but for which we can start the groundwork *now*.

— **Category 3**: Actions that will require strategic or policy changes, which might take some time, so we'd better start our influencing and lobbying *now*.

Note that all three categories demand some action now, even if the results will come later. We find that many traditional action plans are divided into short term, medium term and long term, with the result that many of the medium- and long-term actions are forgotten or ignored. This results in a lack of sustainable change, which in turn leads to the constant revisiting of problems that the team thought were solved ages ago.

CONCLUSION

The principles of good change management are simple. Simple but not easy. We will always be able to find reasons for resorting to directive change, even now we know how ineffective it is. Time will always be short, the demands of the boss for swift action will always be ringing in our ears and opportunities to locate blame or responsibility elsewhere will always be abundant. But we have a genuine opportunity to do it properly. To liberate the creativity and enthusiasm of our team and to improve their working lives and the services we provide. Doing it properly may not be easy but it will turn managing change from a chore to a vocation.

Ask yourself:

➤ Do my team share a vision of how they want things to be?

➤ What qualities do I model as a leader?

➤ Could I give my staff more opportunity to initiate and innovate?

REFERENCES

1 Hellriegel D, Slocum JW, *et al. Organisational Behaviour.* Boston: South Western Publishing; 1998.

2 Sahdev K, Vinnicombe S. *Downsizing and Survivor Syndrome: a study of HR's perception of survivors' responses.* Cranfield: Cranfield University; 1998.

3 Peters T. *Re-imagine.* London: Dorling Kindersley; 2003.

4 Barrett F. Managing and improvising: lessons from jazz. *Career Development International.* 1998; **7**(3): 283–6.

5 Senge P. *The Fifth Discipline: the art and practice of the learning organization.* New York: Doubleday; 1990.

6 Webster B. 'Naked streets are safer, say Tories'. *The Times,* 22 January 2007. Available at www.timesonline.co.uk/tol/news/article1295120.ece (accessed 16 August 2010).

7 Higgs MJ, Rowland D. *Change and Its Leadership: is it time for a change in our thinking?* ECLO Conference. Prague; 2006. (Paper received Academic Award of Merit Distinction.)

8 Hamilton-Baillie B. Streets ahead. *Countryside Voice.* 2005; **Autumn**: 56-7.

9 Kanter R. *The Change Masters.* New York: Simon and Schuster; 1983.

10 Matt. 7.4.

PART 2

Management disciplines

CHAPTER 5

So many meetings!

So far we have looked at how to develop the team as an entity and how to address the unique management and development needs of each member of that team as you bring about change. Much of that work will be carried out in one-to-one discussion with little form and ceremony. However, there are a number of times when good management is on show very publicly. Your reputation as a manager can live or die by the way you organise and run something as routine and common as a meeting, and this whole chapter is dedicated to helping you improve meetings, both for your own reputation and for the mental health of those who attend them!

For many members of the general public, and non-managerial staff inside organisations, a manager's day is assumed to be full of meetings. This may sound okay but a sizeable majority of those people will also view those meetings as irrelevant, longwinded, not real work, avoidance of the real issue, etc. In other words, managers are viewed negatively because they spend so much time on 'unworthy tasks' such as meetings. This perception is all the more damaging because it is largely true. We hear almost daily of managers who have to endure poorly organised and chaired meetings which produce little value compared to the time involved, or who simply copy what they have learned from others and inflict similarly useless meetings on their staff. Such behaviour borders on the criminal and simply provides free ammunition to those who already see the management role as largely unnecessary.

Our view is that meetings are not bad – only *bad* meetings are bad. What do we mean by bad? Take a look at the following list. If your meetings suffer from more than a handful of these symptoms then you have bad meetings on your hands.

➤ A chair that overwhelms and hijacks meetings.
➤ A chair that allows meetings to drift.
➤ A meaningless agenda.
➤ An identical agenda template for every meeting.
➤ No agenda.
➤ Too many long impenetrable papers.

➤ The same old people.
➤ The wrong people.
➤ Recurring issues.
➤ Posturing and politics.
➤ Late arrivers.
➤ Early leavers.
➤ Real decisions that are made outside the meeting.
➤ Endless discussion, revisited at subsequent meetings.
➤ Pointless or irrelevant discussion.
➤ No action.
➤ Insufficent time for the issues at hand.
➤ Discussion which expands to fit the time available.
➤ Not enough business to justify the time and effort.

We often ask participants on our programmes to describe their best and worst meetings, what characterised them and what impact those experiences had on the people involved. While many of the symptoms on the above list crop up time and time again, we are struck by the fact that *all* of them are avoidable and *all* can be influenced by the meeting organiser or chairperson.

So what can you do if your management role involves convening and chairing meetings?

There are three vital stages to consider. These are:

1 decision and purpose.
2 preparation.
3 execution.

DECISION AND PURPOSE

Some of the best meetings are the ones that never happened. This is because someone thought about the issue first and decided that there was no need for the meeting to take place. The first responsibility of a meeting organiser is to make sure that the effort involved is likely to be outweighed by the benefits and if not to postpone the meeting or cancel it outright. This is particularly important for routine meetings that can quickly fall into an automatic pattern and end up being held and attended even if no one really feels it worthwhile. It is almost as if no one is brave enough to call a halt or at least prompt a rethink. If you attend enough of these routine meetings, it is easy to come to view all meetings in the diary as being the same. Even worse, bystanders then associate the people who go to these meetings – i.e. managers – as equally worthless.

Think carefully; what is it about that issue, or issues, that a meeting is best placed to address? What are the alternatives, and how do they stack up? Remember how relieved you are when a meeting you had no interest in attending is cancelled, and think of the other things you could now get on with. Now imagine providing the same gift for others. It could increase respect for you and save everyone some time. Obviously, some could abuse this power to hold or not hold meetings, but on balance it is a risk worth taking because of the appalling experiences some people have of a meeting that served no useful purpose and wasted everyone's time.

Once you are clear about the need for a meeting, produce and publicise a clear and explicit purpose. This will also help you in deciding who should be there. Many of us can recall being invited to a meeting where the general topic was understood but the detailed purpose was not, leading to a situation where either we could not contribute effectively or we were not the most appropriate person to attend. Either way, the outcome was likely to be inconclusive and probably meant another meeting had to be held with the right people. This does not mean that a detailed, formal, bureaucratic, agenda is required for each meeting, but the purpose ought to be more robust and explicit than 'annual leave', 'update on project X', or 'Christmas'. If someone is invited to a hospital-based meeting *'To develop and agree a protocol for admitting violent patients from Accident & Emergency given the latest guidance from the Commission for Health Improvement (summary enclosed)'*, they will know what is expected of them and are far more likely to excuse themselves if it is not the best use of their time. They will be able to nominate a more appropriate person to go or, if they do plan to attend, they can do some thinking beforehand, collect views from colleagues, and then contribute to an informed outcome.

Contrast that with the sheer inability to plan and prepare for a meeting called to *'address the problems of violence in the Emergency Unit'*.

A simple example, you might say, but the absence of this clarity is endemic in some of the organisations with which we work. Even for teams who meet regularly it is just as important to be clear on what the team is there to do and therefore what their meetings are expected to contribute to that purpose.

Some years ago, we were both invited to support an organisation's top management team in its desire to have more effective meetings. During our first encounter we asked what we thought was a simple and uncontentious question – 'What is the team here to do?'. The responses ranged from 'It's obvious, can we move on?', to 'What a stupid question, is that all you management consultants can offer?'. What followed was a messy, unfocused meeting where team members seemed determined to get in the way of progress, often questioning the motives of colleagues as much as the proposals on the table.

When we met with individual team members over the following days and weeks we returned to our earlier 'daft' question. With some of the public bravado now absent, team members were more forthcoming. One person saw the team's purpose as making executive decisions affecting the organisations performance. Someone else saw the team as the place where strategy was developed and blue-sky thinking took place. Yet another team member saw the team meetings as the place where conflict was contained, and a fourth person said honestly that he came along to find out what was going on and to make sure no decisions were made that might compromise his particular department.

In short, we got as many different purposes as there were team members (15) and all but one of those purposes were perfectly legitimate. The problem was that they were different but the differences had not been made explicit, discussed and then reconciled. Therefore each team member came along determined to ensure his or her undisclosed version was achieved, and they actively undermined any discussion that took a different path. It was like watching a 15-direction tug of war, with all of the attendant waste of time, effort and patience. A simple slice of clarity would have helped, but no one was prepared to ask the question 'What are we here for?' Everyone just carried on with, a) the incorrect assumption that they all had the same purpose, and b) a belief that it was just the complexity of the issues that made the meetings difficult.

Even if it done for no other reason than courtesy, it is important that any meeting attendee knows what is expected of them before they arrive, as opposed to finding out too late that they cannot contribute as they would wish.

There are usually three considerations in deciding who needs to be there, and these can apply just as much to the regular routine departmental meeting as to the topical, single issue, project team.

First, one needs to invite those who have a technical contribution to make, and whose absence is likely to compromise the discussion and outcomes. This criterion is not always followed well, and there are plenty of examples of inviting people either based on their rank, or for fear of them feeling left out. If you do not intend to invite someone who, historically, could have expected to be there, speak to them directly and explain your decision rather than leaving them to feel excluded. The latter is more likely to lead to suspicion as to your motives. However, you must feel able to issue invites based on *need* not reputation, otherwise the meeting will end up doing what those present allow it to do.

Second is the mix of people and approaches. If you are setting up a project team that may work together for several months, and meet both formally and informally during that time, then there is merit in gathering a blend of gifts. Chapter 1 looked at the work of Raymond Meredith Belbin and his typology of team roles. This can be a useful way of identifying the right blend of team behaviours, but use it as a framework, not a cage. Do not ignore other helpful behaviours simply because they do not fit Belbin's model perfectly.

The *third* consideration is what we would call the wild-card approach. At times there can be merit in a team or a meeting benefiting from the presence of someone who, on the face of it, has no obvious technical or team-based contribution to make. However, such people may be able to lend extra credibility or gravitas, merely by their power or position in the organisation, or might be able to champion your cause in high places. We make a clear distinction between choosing such people deliberately, and the earlier point about not just inviting people by rank so they don't feel left out. It is normally worth checking this out with the person you propose first so that they do not feel used or end up wasting their time attending something of no interest to them. Used properly this wild-card approach can galvanise a meeting into greater pride and productivity, but if in doubt, stick to the first two criteria.

PREPARATION

You need to do some preparation and you also need to allow others to do the same. You need to think about these sorts of issues:

➤ what you want out of the meeting
➤ who will be there and what they might want
➤ where there is likely to be agreement/disagreement and how extreme you are prepared for the latter to be
➤ should you chair it or not (this can be particularly important if others might see you as the principal beneficiary of the outcome and could therefore accuse you of a conflict of interest)
➤ what information (just enough, not too much or too little) will help those attending to contribute effectively
➤ who you might wish to speak to and *brief* before the meeting, not to stitch things up but to prevent wasting time, especially if there are new arrivals to an otherwise established group who might need bringing up to speed.

If you wish the meeting to be productive, people must know why they are there and be given time to do some thinking beforehand. Many meetings have failed either because the issue, or the need for a decision, came as a surprise to attendees. This leads to decisions being postponed until 'the next meeting' or made in haste with poor information. One piece of good practice that we recommend to many formal management teams and boards is that, if and when there is a need for several complex background papers, each one starts with a very simple summary of the issue, the suggested way forward or recommendation and, most critically, *what it is that the writer is asking the meeting to do*. If the person bringing an item to a meeting (either in paper or verbal form) is not able to articulate what it is they want from others or why it needs to be considered now, how are those others to make a meaningful contribution?

This brings us to the subject of agendas. Does the following style look familiar to you?

MEETING OF THE CORPORATE SUPPORT DIRECTORATE MANAGEMENT TEAM

To be held in the committee room on 15th July, starting at 10.00 a.m.

AGENDA

1 Apologies for absence
2 Minutes of the meeting held on 14th June
3 Matters arising from the minutes
4 Monthly updates from section heads
5 Car parking
6 Forthcoming visit of CEO
7 Health and safety update
8 Holiday shutdown arrangements
9 Financial update
10 Etc.
11 Etc.
12 Any other business
13 Date of next meeting

This style of agenda has been around for years and is responsible for large numbers of bad, useless meetings. There are so many faults with it one hardly knows where to begin but here goes!

1 It is an agenda that almost encourages late arrivals as there is nothing of any significance that will be decided in the first few minutes (and if something is, it can always be unpicked in 'any other business' at the end).
2 The items are in no particular order of importance, which risks a really important issue cropping up right at the end when most people want to leave.
3 It would take a mind reader to work out what is actually required from each item. As a result many of the issues are likely to be discussed for a while and then deferred until next time to allow people to do some thinking.
4 Ill-thought-through items can easily be put on the agenda because there is a meeting coming up, and it allows thinking to be suspended until that meeting.
5 There is a high likelihood that, under item four, section heads will find things to

report for fear of not looking as busy or challenged as their colleagues, thus eating up valuable time.

6 There is no appreciation of how long each item, and therefore the whole meeting, might take, and this makes chairing the meeting almost impossible without being accused of rushing things or of having a hidden agenda.

7 'Any other business' is a ticking bomb and we have all seen the baleful stares of team members towards a colleague who introduces a contentious and complex item just as the end of the meeting was in sight. In such circumstances it is almost certain that either the issue will be deferred until next time, or a hasty and instantly regretted decision will be made in the last few minutes.

Need we go on?

Most meetings do not really need the highly formalised structure of apologies, minutes, matters arising, followed by 15 unrelated items and concluding with 'any other business' and date of next meeting. In fact these agendas can get in the way of productive meetings and are one of the symptoms of routine, process-driven and frustrating experiences. In contrast, there are three vital components of a useful agenda. They are:

1 clarity of items and their purpose
2 linking of associated items
3 a match between time and content.

An agenda item simply containing words such as 'car parking', 'Christmas', 'rotas', 'new department' and 'HR policies' is wholly inadequate and will leave the chair of the meeting with the unenviable tasks of either spending valuable time finding out the purpose, or replacing each person's individual interpretation of that item with the real one. Good practice is for each item to have some explanation of the specific issue and what is required.

You may have been in meetings where the outcome of the discussion of a later item requires a reopening of discussion on an earlier topic. This is usually evidence of an agenda that has been put together as the items came in with little analysis or discernment. One way to avoid this problem, as well as the likelihood that awkward issues crop up near the end when everyone has had enough or when some have already left, is to structure the agenda as follows.

Don't be fooled by the apparent simplicity of this approach – it can and will transform your meetings.

Section 1   Items requiring a *decision* today.
Section 2   Items calling for *discussion* today (with decisions taken later).
Section 3   Items for *information* and note.

Here is an example of an agenda that follows that structure.

MEETING OF THE DESIGN TEAM OF BLOGGS PLC

To be held on Tuesday 28 February in HQ Meeting Room 4,
between 10 a.m. and 11:30 a.m.

AGENDA

Items for decision today

1   Proposed merger with Smith and Sons PLC (Jim Barnes).
    To agree the arrangements for transferring employment of existing staff and endorse
    the proposed redundancy package set out in JB's paper (attached).
2   Financial report (Sue Smith).
    To agree project income targets for the 1st and 2nd quarters of next year given the
    outturn indicated in the latest financial report.
3   Major risk analysis (Manager Dept B).
    To approve the proposed changes to risk assessments as outlined in Dept B's
    monthly report (pages 2 and 3).

Items for discussion

4   Review of training (Andy Chard).
    To generate ideas for improving the uptake of training course places in the light of
    the review of training circulated to members last month.

Items for information

5   Car parking – to note the closure of the north car park during March for building
    works.
6   Update on Project Firefly – to note the completion of phase 4 and the compliments
    from the client (see attached letter).
7   Minutes of the quality sub-group – to receive these minutes and note the reductions
    in waste processes.
8   Departmental reports – to note contents and key events (more info direct from
    authors).
    Dept A
    Dept B
    Dept C
9   Date of next meeting – 29th March.

This approach requires that any person wanting to raise an item at the meeting
(including the person chairing the meeting) *has to be clear* why they are raising it,
what they need from the participants and therefore which part of the agenda it
fits within. By stating a clear purpose for each item on the agenda, and by ensuring

that any supporting paper is brief, succinct and designed to help participants do what is asked of them, the meeting will flow better, will be easier to chair, will be shorter and will lead to fewer items being deferred due to lack of notice. Just as importantly, it will lead to fewer items making it onto the agenda as people find better ways of getting the business done.

Its other benefits are that it prevents the important items being dealt with last, and that it allows both proposer and attendee to be clear about what is expected. In the event of time running out, the less critical information items can be dropped, or dealt with in other ways. More subtly it can 'train' people to be on time, as they will know that the key decisions are to be made first.

We not only use this approach with our own meetings, we have received unanimously positive feedback from other managers about the transformational impact this approach has on their meetings. Typically they report a significant reduction in meeting length, greater motivation and attendance, higher quality discussion, fewer late arrivals and more sustainable decision-making.

One useful tactic to help with the timing of meetings is to allocate an estimated time for each item. Of course it can only be an estimate and it would be a foolish chairperson that abruptly halted a discussion just when agreement was within grasp, simply because the allotted time had expired. However, it can be a useful gauge of the relative importance of issues, and an astute chairman can use the timings as a pacing tool by reminding the meeting how long they either have for this item, or how long they have been discussing it. Self-evidently, if the estimated time accumulates to more than the time available, the chair has to either revise the timings or prune the agenda.

RUNNING (CHAIRING) THE MEETING: CONTENT AND PROCESS

Whilst there will be some who would prefer, and exploit, a weak chairperson, most meeting goers appreciate professional chairing. You, along with everyone else at the meeting, have plenty of other things to do, and so chairing a businesslike, focused, outcome-led meeting is a mark of courtesy to all present.

Any meeting consists of content (what is done) and process (the way it is done). A good chair has to keep an eye on both.

Process issues include:

➤ When and where should the meeting be held?
➤ How should the meeting be conducted? (formal/informal, chaired/facilitated, etc.)
➤ How can it be ensured that every member is allowed to contribute?
➤ How much time is needed?

Content issues include:
➤ What information is needed for a good decision to be made?
➤ What needs to be discussed, decided or noted?

One way of understanding the process part of the chairing role is to compare it to the work of a sports referee.

A good referee is someone who makes it clear to all parties what the rules are (the markings on the pitch), sets the ball in play, upholds the rules, marks a goal by blowing a whistle and brings play back to the centre to start again.

A good chair makes the rules clear (the agenda), sets the ball in play (introduces an item or a presenter), upholds the rules (invites contributions and intervenes where inappropriate comments are made), marks a goal (confirms a decision) and brings play back to the centre (moves to the next item).

Of course the analogy is flawed in that a referee is uninterested in the performance or result but it can be a helpful way of seeing the chair as being concerned with the process as much as with the content of the meeting. It is worth noting that in a good game no one really notices the referee – he or she lets the game flow because everyone knows the rules and just gets on with it. Good meetings are the same.

DOING THINGS DIFFERENTLY

In most organisations there is an unspoken but persistent belief that meetings have to take place around a table where the chair leads the members through a list of things to talk about while someone writes minutes. In some cases this is an entirely appropriate way to conduct business. In others it is actually counterproductive. Imagine the purpose of the meeting is to generate ideas. Not everyone likes to do their thinking out loud in a large group – so maybe you need to give people enough notice so they can come with ideas at the ready, or perhaps part of the meeting could be spent in smaller discussion groups. This will almost certainly lead to more ideas. Some people find it helpful to doodle as they think, so perhaps you could provide paper and pens. A relaxed, even playful mood can often help people to think creatively but the linear way of thinking and talking that formal meetings and agendas tend to promote will squash, rather than release, creativity. The key here is that form should follow function. Particularly where you want people to be imaginative, honest or receptive, you should consider whether the traditional boardroom/agenda/chairperson approach would help or hinder. Here are some examples of doing things differently.
➤ At a meeting to consider long-term strategy in a team facing many challenges, internal and external, I asked the members to work in small groups to draw how they saw the future. The images varied from a broken-down car at a crossroads to a futuristic metropolis. The discussion that followed was honest

and fruitful. Using images had helped the group express not only their professional concerns but also their personal anxieties. Not only this but we reached this point of honesty and realism far quicker than if we had conducted the meeting formally.

➤ I once attended a meeting held to critique a new policy being considered by an NHS organisation. The person leading the meeting asked each of us to consider the policy from the perspective of a group of people who would be affected by it. Depending on the perspective we were allocated, we were challenged to imagine how a patient, or staff member, or taxpayer might see what we were proposing to do. As a result, our critique of the draft policy was much more rigorous and well rounded.

➤ At a large staff meeting held to consult on a new management structure, I gave each person a pad of sticky notes. I then put up four pieces of flip-chart paper, one in each corner of the room. One had the title 'hopes', another was headed 'fears', the title of the third was 'bridges' and the fourth 'barriers'. I invited people to write down as many thoughts as possible about:
— hopes: their hopes for the new structure
— fears: their anxieties
    bridges: things that would promote a smooth transition
— barriers: things that could get in the way.

I then asked them to put their sticky notes on the appropriate flip chart. This enabled a much greater number and diversity of comments than the 'question and answer' format often used for this kind of meeting. The anonymity allowed by this method may also have helped people express themselves more honestly. I was then able to sort people's comments into themes that guided the rest of the consultation process.

Our point here is not that drawing or role-playing is always better than simply talking. What we are arguing for is a meeting *process* that is thoughtfully chosen to satisfy the purpose of each specific meeting.

TIPS FOR CHAIRING A MEETING

A number of tips can make the difference between good and bad chairing.

➤ Start on time. Your failure to do so legitimises future late arrivals. This does mean *you* have to be there on time!

➤ Ensure all present are clear on the purpose and time period of the meeting. If some genuinely have to leave early then find that out at the start rather than being surprised by their embarrassed exit.

➤ If papers for items have already been circulated, do not allow the authors to simply repeat their contents. Always assume that people have read the papers

– let them admit that they haven't rather than waste everyone's time with unnecessary presentations. Draw the meeting's attention to the paper, and the action required, invite the speaker to add anything of substance emerging since the paper was produced and to emphasise any critical factor, and then invite a response. Remember the response should be commensurate with the reason why the item was on the agenda in the first place, so be prepared to curtail interesting but irrelevant discussion.

➤ Continue to invite contributions and watch for the quieter ones being drowned out by the more vocal attendees. Do not embarrass the former by putting them on the spot, but do not close an item before asking again whether *anyone else* has a view not yet expressed.

➤ Revisit the purpose of the item and ask whether the decision or recommend-ation is confirmed. If it is, quickly seek clarity on what will happen next and then move on. If the answer is no, push for agreement as to how the issue will now be handled. Do not leave issues hanging in the air, for these loose ends tend to dominate the *matters arising* part of a subsequent meeting.

➤ Dealing with distractions is the chairperson's responsibility. If you feel that mobile phones should be on silent, or off, say so at the start. If a couple of people start their own private meeting, intervene firmly but politely by asking whether they have anything to add to what is being said. Some chairs use the phrase 'one meeting at a time please' to achieve the same effect.

➤ Never 'take on' anyone from the chair. It is an abuse of the position and far from reassuring other members, may make them uneasy in case they are next in line. If you have to tackle one person about their behaviour, call for a quick recess and deal with them in private. The same tactic can be used if the meeting is moving beyond creative tension and is becoming overheated. Remember the chairman is the caretaker of process and the injection of a bit of process can help diffuse tensions. Joining in the argument from the chair, particularly at high volume, simply reduces the meeting to a state of anarchy.

➤ If you feel that your personal and professional contribution to a meeting is so important to you that you must be free of other duties, seek another chair for the meeting. That is not to say a chair can never express an opinion, but you need to think through how you would be perceived if, as chair, you refused to yield on a controversial issue.

➤ Finish on time or before. A late finish for one meeting is likely to increase the number of early departures at the next one, as people are not confident that they will be away 'on time'. If, unavoidably, more time is needed, ask the members whether they would prefer to postpone other agenda items or carry on.

➤ It is good practice, every so often, to conclude the meeting with a quick review of how it went, and whether people feel that changes should be considered. This can prevent a regular or routine meeting from becoming stale, and may allow the issue of change of membership to be safely discussed.

➤ If minutes are required, make them appropriate to the needs of the meeting. Most people are comfortable with action points rather than fully minuted and attributed discussions. If possible do not take the minutes yourself as it can be both distracting from the role and may introduce a conflict of interest. Whichever way they are done, they should not be circulated until you have seen them and satisfied yourself that they reflect the essence of the meeting.

One of our clients was the management board of a health-commissioning organisation where executive and non-executive directors came together on a bimonthly basis to hold its meetings in public. They wanted some help with board development and part of this involved looking at their meeting processes. At one of the meetings we observed an example of well-intentioned but poor chairmanship, which led to an almost complete disengagement by the non-executives present.

As might be expected from a publicly accountable body, there were a large number of serious issues, all of which were supported by long and complicated reports, with each one being 'presented' by its relevant executive director. After each presentation the chairman had a habit of summarising the key issues as he saw them, added his own research and opinions and made it clear what he thought ought to happen next. As soon as he finished speaking, the CEO would wade in and, in a genuine attempt to be helpful, would recount the meetings and conversations she had had with key officials, all of which supported the chairman's suggestions. At which point the chairman would finally throw the item open for discussion. You can imagine how engaged the rest of the team were by then. It seemed clear that one either agreed with the chairman (verbally or by staying silent) or challenged the system and got a reputation for being difficult. Several non-executives told us afterwards that it was simply not worth prolonging the discussion but they felt most unhappy with the whole experience.

Bear in mind this was not a cunning attempt by the chair and CEO to stifle debate, they genuinely thought they were helping.

The moral of the story is that once the main issues are on the table, the chair should look after the process and be the last to offer a personal opinion, unless there are clearly some non-negotiables that need to be stated upfront.

CHAPTER 6

Making confident presentations

At some time in their careers managers will need to stand (or sit) in front of a group and make a presentation. To go into management thinking that this can be avoided is both delusional and risks losing you opportunities to represent your team or service. For some of us our first formal presentation was a proud rite of passage, for others it was about as welcome and enjoyable as a visit to the dentist. Whatever your experience of presentations, they continue to play a central role in how organisations communicate within and between themselves. Those of us who now make part of our living from standing in front of groups are always in danger of forgetting or underestimating the excitement and anxiety that making a presentation can invoke, and what makes the subject even more emotive is that people's common experience of presentations is less than positive. It seems that, paradoxically, while it is a powerful way of communicating and influencing others, it is regularly done badly.

In a society obsessed by information, imagery and the need for speed in everything (from ordering a burger to getting to the heart of a complex problem), the demand for punchy, image-rich, zappy, high-impact presentations has unwittingly raised the performance bar. This has left occasional presenters feeling unsure as to how to respond and what technology to use. The result in many organisations is that PowerPoint is no longer just an optional tool – it is either compulsory or, at the very least, the norm. Indeed, those who prefer not to use this particular method of presenting often report that their motives and competence are questioned, or that less value is placed on their work.

In one organisation we consult to, copies of PowerPoint slides are used as the agenda and papers for meetings, and as an aide-memoire for those who couldn't be there. Without in any way criticising the concept and potential uses of this presentation medium, the current obsession with PowerPoint risks reducing every issue to a handful of bullet points and leaving non-users feeling second class.

In this chapter we will look at the whole concept of presentations: their purpose, how to plan an effective presentation, how to manage yourself and your audience on the day and how to use the various tools to add value to your presentation. PowerPoint can make a valuable contribution to this process and we will demonstrate its benefits and drawbacks with equal clarity. However, there will also be plenty of advice for those who cannot, or choose not to, use computer-based technology to aid their presentations.

When we cover this topic in our Vital Signs programme, participants are asked to identify examples of good and poor presentations in their recent memory. As you might expect, many of the aspects of poor presentations are the opposite of those found in the better ones but the sorts of examples generated for *good* presentations included:

➤ meeting the audience's needs
➤ demonstrating competence and credibility (being thoroughly prepared and in control of the material)
➤ sounding interested and interesting
➤ good eye contact
➤ answering the *'Why are we here?'* question quickly
➤ not being fazed by questions and interruptions
➤ having a clear purpose and sticking to it
➤ finishing on time or early
➤ using any technology to add to the presentation rather than to complicate or confuse
➤ no contradiction between what is being said and what is being shown on screen
➤ if using slides, making sure they are simple and legible.

In contrast, the ingredients of *poor* presentations included:
➤ trying to cram too much information into a short time
➤ not being clear as regards the purpose
➤ not getting to the point quickly
➤ uninspiring voice and body language
➤ distracting habits
➤ cluttered and illegible slides (in PowerPoint or when using overhead acetates)
➤ reading slides verbatim (and so turning their back on the audience while doing so)
➤ not handling questions well or at all
➤ not looking prepared
➤ appearing blasé

➤ lacking confidence in the technology (if used)
➤ reading from a script.

It is interesting to note that none of the examples produced by participants cite personal nervousness as a *primary* contributor to poor presentations. This is because we recognise it is natural for people to experience some anxiety when entering what is for many an unusual environment. If the subject is important, and if the views of the audience are equally so, any presenter worth their salt should be 'up for it' and their performance is likely to be sharpened by a degree of apprehensiveness. Indeed many famous and respected actors admit to being so affected by stage fright that they are physically sick beforehand. However, they would also argue that this physiological reaction actually helps them focus and do their jobs better.

Therefore anxiety in itself need not be a barrier to making effective presentations, and most human beings will have a modicum of sympathy and support for fledging presenters who work through their nerves. After all they have been there themselves!

> I once heard someone say that they still get butterflies in their stomach before a major event but they have *trained them to fly in formation*. I think that is a wonderful metaphor for the tools we are about to cover in this section. They work with your natural anxiety but help you to put those butterflies to good use.

Before we move on to look at how to approach the process of planning and then delivering an effective presentation, one final reminder about the importance of getting it right. Poor presentations tend to produce two negative outcomes.
➤ First, they tend to weaken the argument or case being put forward and make it easy for an audience to disengage or say no. This is particularly true if the struggle of the presenter becomes more interesting than the topic and leads to the audience being distracted.
➤ Second, and more damaging in the longer term, a poor presentation weakens the personal credibility of the presenter so that next time the same audience is almost conditioned to expect a poor experience.

Both of these outcomes can be a tad unjustified, particularly if the presenter is only doing what they think best (probably with no training or support) or the audience itself is being a little unprofessional. However, it makes sense to get it right first time, every time, and the following advice will be useful to both new and experienced presenters alike.

Our advice is set out in three parts – preparation, technology and delivery.

PREPARATION

Let us start with the trigger for most presentations – either you are asked to make a presentation to a meeting or a group, or you actually request the time and space to make a presentation. The event might be a management meeting, a conference, a seminar, an informal get together of your own department or even a job interview.

There are six essential issues to tackle up front, each of which will be explained further in a moment.

1 You need to be clear in your mind that a presentation (by which we mean physically being in front of a group of people and having a set time to communicate an issue or proposal to them) is the best way of achieving the outcome you desire.

2 Having established that a presentation is the most effective medium, make sure that you are the right person, or that you will be by the time the presentation takes place.

3 Make sure you have mastery of the material you are about to present, and of any technology/visual aids you will be using.

4 Carry out some research into your audience – who they are, what their interests are, what information or approach they tend to prefer.

5 Make sure that you and your audience has the same understanding of why they and you are going to be in the same room at the same time.

6 You need to actually plan the flow of the presentation, making sure you get attention, get to the point quickly, cover the essentials rather than the fripperies and conclude crisply and with authority.

More detail on each of these points follows.

Is a presentation the best method?

As we argued earlier, presentations, particularly those using PowerPoint, have fast become the expected way of communicating to meetings and other events. But are they always the best way? Of course if others have asked you to present, or it is a requirement for a job interview, then your room for manoeuvre is more limited, but in all other situations ask yourself whether there are other communication methods that might be more cost effective in achieving the same result. Those methods might include:

➤ a series of one-to-one discussions (more time consuming certainly, but they may reveal support or objections that a formal presentation might not uncover)

➤ writing a discussion paper and giving people time to respond as they see fit

➤ talking to just the relevant person and not wasting everyone else's time on an irrelevant monologue, etc.

Even if coming to a group with ideas is the best way it still does not follow that a formal stand-up technology-based presentation is required. I have vivid memories of working with some groups where they have positively welcomed me coming with more of a 'fireside chat' approach to the presentation, in contrast to their constant diet of PowerPoint and images. Frankly there are some issues that will benefit from simply pulling up a chair and saying something like: *'There are three issues affecting our performance at present (cue holding up three fingers of one hand) – they are a, b and c. I intend to quickly summarise these and my proposal for the way forward. Then I would really appreciate your views.'*

What this approach tends to do is introduce a level of humanity and intimacy that formal presentations sometimes lack and it seems to draw the audience into the process. In contrast, formal presentations can almost encourage the audience to sit back, adopt a passive stance and wait to be impressed.

Make sure you are the right person

Whether we are made anxious by the request or not, there is always a sense of flattery when asked to present. Someone thinks you have a valuable role to play and that your ideas are worth listening to. Hang on to this positive thought – it will be useful later on. However, being asked and saying yes are two different things. If you do not think you are the right person, perhaps because there are others in the team who possess a greater expertise or perhaps because those others may just be able to communicate the issues in a language the audience will quickly understand, it will be in your best interests to ask others to step in. Just to be quite clear here, we are not advocating avoidance. In fact, if you remember the intrinsic motivating factors we covered in Chapter 2, it could significantly enhance the value of a colleague's job if *they* get a chance to communicate on a stage normally reserved for more senior staff. Therefore if your assessment is that there are others better placed, and your motives are pure, then politely decline and give others their opportunity to shine.

If we assume that you are the right person, you need to make sure that this faith in your ability is justified on the day. This means that you need to prepare, research, rehearse, and most importantly, *believe* that you have a right to be there and that the audience needs your expertise. Many an otherwise good presentation has been spoiled by an almost apologetic presenter who starts the session by openly questioning why they have been asked and saying 'I hope that you find some of this useful'. After such an underwhelming introduction why should the audience be the slightest bit interested?

Mastery of the material and the technology

Our years of presenting and listening to others present has simply confirmed that those who talk with crisp and jargon-free authority about a subject they know well make better, more confident presentations than those who come unprepared and try to wing it on the day.

There is no substitute for being familiar with:

➤ your material
➤ the proposal you are putting forward
➤ the alternatives
➤ the evidence.

One way to test yourself before the big day is to ruthlessly look for the weaknesses in your argument and imagine yourself responding to those challenges. Better still, ask someone who is not as immersed in the issue as you are and not as biased. They may not be able to give an expert opinion but they are still likely to spot the obvious flaws. Even their naïve questions about your material may well expose some faulty thinking, jargon or issues you may have taken for granted. Bear in mind that being comfortable with the material is not the same as memorising a script.

> The problem with a script is that it almost hems you in on the day and forces you to cover things in the set order. As soon as a question or challenge requires you to go 'off script' it can be difficult to find your way back later. Reading from a script also changes your speech delivery, flattens out all of the rise and fall in your voice, and completely breaks eye contact with your audience. We cover the alternatives to having a script later.

Once you are in control of the data, the arguments and the counter-arguments, you can turn your attention to what technology might help and how to make it all work.

We have much more comprehensive advice later on how to use technology such as PowerPoint, as well as the less complex alternatives, but for now it is enough to stress that you must not go into any presentation environment without being completely confident with what you are using the technology for, how it works and what to do if it goes wrong on the day. We normally advise managers to get so confident with the material that even if the technology went AWOL on the day or failed to work, they could still deliver the main points without compromise. In this way the technology becomes what it should always be – a tool, not a crutch.

Researching the audience

We remain surprised and concerned at the large number of managers who find themselves delivering important presentations to a group of virtual strangers, without bothering to find out a few essential facts beforehand. Not only is this discourteous to the audience, it leaves the presenter at real risk of missing the target (in terms of both the message and the medium).

If I am asked to give any presentation there are vital pieces of information I need beforehand. These are:

➤ who will be there, their jobs, and their areas of interest
➤ the group's preference for types of information (big ideas/lots of detail/ options/one precise plan, etc.)
➤ if it is a longer meeting at which I am presenting one item, I need to know what topic is just before/after mine and whether it will involve lots of detailed slides.

Some of this information is easy to obtain just by getting hold of previous agendas/ minutes. If there are still gaps it is always a good idea to ring the chair of the meeting and politely state that in order to meet the group's needs it would help to be prepared. Once you have this information use it to fine-tune the detail of your presentation.

For example, if the group wants and attaches great importance to detailed evidence and data, it makes no sense to breeze in and try to sell a broad vision or big idea. Conversely a group that needs a clear plan will not be impressed by vague strategies and light-touch monitoring arrangements. In practice you will find most groups have a mixture of preferences and so you will have to cover all the bases in your presentation.

Information gathered on the structure and flow of the meeting you are attending can help you decide whether to make the presentation lighter or more serious. As a general rule I would normally follow on from a heavy, 'data-rich' item by keeping my item light, direct and to the point. Audiences like that attention to their needs.

Ensuring everyone's understanding of the item is the same

This is so obvious that it is often taken for granted or ignored. The time to find out exactly what a group is asking for is before you start! To find out halfway through that what you are covering is not what was required or expected risks both irritating the group and damaging your own reputation. If they have asked you to present something, do not say yes until you have complete clarity. Similarly if you have requested time at the group's meeting make sure that the agenda item is worded to your satisfaction. Refer to the section on agendas in Chapter 5 for more advice on the working of agenda items.

Planning the presentation itself

Here we are talking about how you order your material for the day, not how you go about researching the topic or putting together the evidence you need to support the proposal you are making.

Common problems caused by a lack of planning include:

➤ trying to pack too much material (slides, arguments, data, evidence, etc.) into the time available, which risks overrunning or gabbling to try and finish on time

➤ not being clear on the central argument, which risks confusing or disengaging the audience

➤ not starting *and* ending with clarity and confidence, which risks the audience associating your lack of impact with the quality of your case.

One way of overcoming these problems is to use a simple structure for the planning process. It has three components.

1 The first step is to start from your end point and work back. This seems coun-terintuitive but is highly effective. It involves consciously thinking through your closing remarks, as if you were actually in the room giving your presentation. What would you be saying as you summarise your case and invite questions? Here is an imaginary but realistic 'closing statement':

> *So to summarise, you are already aware of the current problem of missed appoint-ments in the outpatient department. These are currently costing the organisation £250k a year and causing us to miss critical performance targets. You asked me to research some solutions and the most suitable of these is to text those patients who have mobile phones, two days prior to their appointments. This would cost £15k a year in texts and training, but would save over £230k annually. I could have the system in place within two weeks if you can agree to the proposal today. I would be happy to take questions.*

In practice you might not end up using each and every word, but that is not the point of the exercise. The main purpose is to remind you of the key points of your presentation, without padding or deviation. If you cannot create this clos-ing statement it is possibly due to a lack of mastery of the material or perhaps the central message of the presentation is still unclear.

2 Once you have this crisp and clear closing statement, you can use it to set the scene at the start. We have already mentioned that some poor presentations start with a whimper and fail to either set the scene or grab the attention of the audi-ence. Unless you can quickly answer the audience's unspoken question, 'Why should I listen to this?', you will swiftly lose their interest. Therefore, without being gratuitously dramatic or exaggerating the issue, it is vital that you get to the point quickly. An edited version of your closing statement is an excellent way of achieving a powerful and influential start. Using our fictitious example above, I could say:

Thank you for asking me to present to you today. As you know the missed appointments in outpatients are a major problem and I bring to you today a cost-effective solution. At present these missed appointments cost us £250k per year, and are in breach of the national targets, but I have researched a tried and tested solution whereby we text patients a few days before their appointment. This will save far more than it costs and can be implemented within weeks. Over the next few minutes I will outline the size of the problem, the various options, why we chose the texting option and what it will cost. I will then seek your approval to proceed.

You will note that all the main elements of the closing remarks are here in the introduction, but not repeated parrot fashion. Using the wording above, no one in the audience will be in any doubt what is being presented, why and what they are expected to do in response. If you read the words out loud, they will take less than 60 seconds to say, well within the attention span of even the most weary audience member.

3   If you now look at your opening and closing statements, what should be clear are the critical few issues that need to be covered in the presentation. In other words the structure will emerge from the statements and you can use that structure to plan the middle part of the presentation. As you do so the whole presentation will hang together, flow logically and, most importantly, it will be mercifully free of padding, side issues, distractions and waffle. Our experience of such an approach to presentations is that it greatly improves the clarity and impact of the message, it encourages greater audience engagement, and it leads to shorter presentations. It should be pointed out that if the case you are arguing is poor then no amount of good structure will save it, but if the underlying case is good, this approach will give it the best opportunity to shine

On our Vital Signs programme we ask our participants to use this method to construct and deliver a 2-minute pitch, on a real and pressing issue. Without exception they report being surprised at how much they can cover in those 2 minutes, simply by being clear throughout on the main message and being ruthless in stripping away the trimmings. If this is what can be achieved in 2 minutes, imagine the luxury of having 10 or 15 minutes! No more overrunning, plenty of time for questions and discussion and an audience that has its needs met quickly and clearly.

This approach is journalistic rather than academic and you can see it being successfully utilised in newspapers, news programmes and movie trailers. We are given the headlines, then the main issues are unpacked and then there is a summary of the headlines. It also mirrors the advice given to trainers – 'tell 'em what you're going to tell 'em, tell 'em, then tell 'em what you've told 'em'.

TECHNOLOGY

In this context we are using the word technology very broadly to describe any external device (flip chart, overhead projector, PowerPoint, props, etc.) that you feel will add value to your presentation.

The phrase 'add value' is critical here. We are not talking about 'livening up' an otherwise dull presentation; any diversion away from you and the words you are using must add something unique and vital, otherwise it risks actually distracting the audience and weakening your message.

The phrase 'form follows function' is crucial to your choice of technology (if any). You need to look hard at the purpose of the presentation, the subject matter, the importance of any data, the complexity of the subject, the needs of your audience (covered earlier) and your own comfort levels, and then, and only then, choose the appropriate medium for delivering that message. The following (Table 7.1) is intended as general guidance only, and ultimately you must make your own judgement.

TABLE 7.1 Types of technology

Type of technology	Appropriate uses
None	The subject is highly personal and emotive
	The audience have previously expressed dissatisfaction at the overuse of slides
	You want to engage the audience in dialogue right from the start and throughout
	The time limit is so short it would take longer to set the technology up than it would to deliver the message
Flip chart (created during the presentation)	Informal situations such as small team seminars, training workshops and strategy timeouts
	When the key messages need to emerge from the discussion and need to be captured immediately
	When you want to highlight key words and then connect them as the presentation goes on (with lines, circles and arrows, etc.)
	When you want the presentation to look intuitive and organic
Flip chart (pre-prepared)	When clarity is required but the audience is not equipped for, or not used to, PowerPoint
	When you want a more homely feel or want to tell a personal story (handwriting seems to convey humanity!)
PowerPoint	When communicating facts, figures and clear arguments

(*continued*)

Type of technology	Appropriate uses
Powerpoint (*cont*)	When demonstrating the complexity of an issue by building up a diagram piece by piece When showing the dynamics of an issue (by judicious use of the moving graphics capability) For displaying images/photos/maps

POWERPOINT

To conclude this section on technology, a few pieces of advice about using PowerPoint, the medium often handled less well than the others.'

Common PowerPoint problems (some of which have been mentioned earlier) include:

➤ over packing of slides (reducing both legibility and impact)

➤ endless lists (with each point revealing one by one)

➤ presenter being 'controlled' by the order of slides (and using them solely as prompts for their message).

All three can be eliminated completely by the use of a few simple tips. We should stress that this is not intended as a complete manual on using PowerPoint. Many excellent publications are available and anyone thinking of using this medium on a regular basis is advised to obtain a reputable technical guide.

First, slide design, using bullet points as one example. Bullet points are a common feature in PowerPoint slides and used correctly are an efficient way of getting information across. However, they tend to lead to a reductionist approach whereby almost everything is explained in bullet-point form, and the endless bullet-point reveals can eat up time at an alarming pace. If bullet points are what you want, there are three main design options.

➤ *The basic reveal*, where each item appears in turn, normally as a result of a mouse or keyboard click. This is really useful if you want to keep your audience fixed on the point you are discussing and not racing ahead to look at the rest of the list. Keep the numbers of points small (four to six) otherwise it gets tedious, and time consuming. Why not include the number of points in the title of the slide (e.g. '5 Problem Areas', or '4 Main Options') so that the audience can see how the process is going?

➤ *The big picture*, where all points appear at once (this is the default way PowerPoint shows bullet points). The main use of this approach is, as the name suggests, when you want to show the big picture, demonstrate the breadth or scope of an issue or where you need to show all the facets of a project/issue. The key here is not to go through each one in turn. It is normally enough to prepare the audience (e.g. 'As you will now see, this project has more components than most people previously thought.') Put up the list, pause and let people read it for themselves. The impact is in that bigger picture, not the detail, and if you start to go through each one you will bore the audience, most of whom will probably be wondering why you are helping them read, or skipping to another point further down your list.

➤ *The managed big picture*, where all the points appear at once, but then some are highlighted for special attention. This way of showing points is really good for demonstrating both a breadth of knowledge *and* an acknowledgement that time is short so we must concentrate on the priority areas. The simplest way of doing this is to copy the original slide and then place the points you do want to major on in bold type or a different colour. If you say something like 'As you can see, there is much to do in this project, but in view of the time today and the particular needs of this group I intend to concentrate on these three', you will save valuable time while still giving the impression you know about all the issues.

Again, see a technical guide for how to create these sorts of slides. The names we have given these designs are ours, but the manuals will show you how to achieve these effects.

The key is to make sure you use the right approach for the job at hand. Even if PowerPoint is compulsory in your organisation there is still room for you to use different approaches and your presentations will stand out from the crowd if you do.

Please note that our references to PowerPoint apply equally to other proprietry software such as open source products or Apple's Keynote application.

Now for some simple tools to show that you are in charge of the equipment and not vice versa; essential if you want the audience to concentrate on your message not your struggle with the kit.

If you want the audience to come back and focus their whole attention on you for a while (perhaps before going on to a new topic or when responding to questions), blank the screen. On most laptops this can be done by simply pressing the B or W key once. As you might have guessed, B turns the screen black whereas W makes it go white. Pressing either key again turns the screen back on where you left it. One of the benefits of this tool is that it prevents any audience confusion as to whether they should be listening to you or looking at something, particularly if what is on the slide is not what you are explaining at that time. It is also far more professional than trying to cover up the projector lens or shutting down the presentation and having to turn it on again later.

Always use slide numbers (see the manuals for advice on how and where to put them on the slide). The first benefit is that it will guard against you creating too many slides for the time available. We normally advise presenters against using more than four or five slides in a 10-minute presentation, otherwise the tendency will be to rush through them or overrun. Having the slide numbers show up as you sit at your desk doing the planning will prevent you from just hitting the 'new slide' button without thinking.

The second and rather cool benefit of slide numbers is that you can use them to navigate directly to a slide during your presentation. You just type in that slide number on your keyboard, press enter or return and 'hey presto' that slide appears instantly. No more feverish pressing of the up and down arrow with the audience watching all the other slides and complex builds flash in front of their eyes. It is much more professional to simply go direct, whether in response to a question, in order to re-emphasise an earlier point, or just to skip to the end slide if time is running out. It demonstrates you are in command and can help to reassure the audience as to the credibility of your proposal.

DELIVERY

So, you are ready. The preparation has been done, the research carried out and the material mastered. The rehearsals have gone well and you know you can finish within the time limit given. The technology (where appropriate) has been tested and everything is in place. Wait a minute, what's that in your hand? A script? Stop right there.

As we mentioned earlier a script can cause your voice to flatten out and lose all the passion and commitment you might feel towards your topic. It can also break eye contact, remove all flexibility and spontaneity and, if all you were going to do was read out a script, why did you not send an email instead and save everybody some time? The final drawback of a script is that it is often a big piece of paper to hold, and any hand movements you might make naturally will be exaggerated by the A4 paper and could distract the audience.

A far better alternative is to use small notecards (sometimes called flash cards), the size of postcards, on which you can put key words and phrases to keep you on track and remind you of the main points. You can also give yourself reminders such as 'look up', 'smile', 'pause', 'slow down', 'five minutes gone?'. Make sure you number the cards and link them together using those green 'treasury tags' so that if they fall to the floor they will stay in the right order.

Right, *now* you are ready. A few tips will keep you in control and looking professional during the presentation itself.

➤ *Start confidently.* Do not waffle and creep into the topic. Don't use humour unless you are really sure of your material and the audience, as jokes 'to warm things up' often fall flat and the embarrassing silence simply adds more pressure. Look up, engage a few pairs of eyes and get attention right away. The planning tool we gave you earlier will help to give your opening statements real impact.

➤ Let the audience know the *overall structure* of the presentation right at the start and then stick to it. At the end of each section, summarise and mark the change to the next part. If you have time, and don't mind questions as you go along, you might want to signal this change by asking if there are 'any questions before we move on?'. If you are tight for time, let the audience know at the start that you will be happy to take questions at the end and then be gentle but firm in the face of any interruptions.

➤ *Eye contact* is essential if you are to justify actually being in the same room as your audience! Do not stare at anyone; just move your eyes from one part of the room to another in a fairly random and relaxed way, not forgetting to include those on either side of the room who might otherwise feel excluded. There is no need to look like a radar device, tracking round the room in a circular motion. Make it natural and your approach will then blend into the background and not distract the audience.

➤ *Pause.* You may have limited time for your presentation but if the whole session is a constant stream of words, images and data, even the most intelligent and focused audience will be overwhelmed. If you know there is a critical part of your presentation, make sure you pause immediately afterwards to let the point sink in. If using PowerPoint, letting the audience take in a complex slide or read a key statement for themselves allows you to pause, take a sip of water, check your notes and then move on. The rhythm of a presentation can be as influential as the content.

➤ *If you lose your place,* do not bluff or waffle. Just state calmly 'Excuse me a moment, I've lost my train of thought', check your notes and then pick up where you left off. This will be less likely if you use notecards, but audiences are human too – they have been where you are – and it is how you recover that will be remembered.

➤ If using PowerPoint, *position the laptop in front of you* and ensure it is easy to see at a glance. By default most laptops are configured to show the same slide on the screen as is being projected onto the wall behind you. The various manuals will help if your laptop does not behave that way. You can then reassure yourself that the right slide/topic is on the screen and it prevents you from having to turn round to check (which can break contact with your audience and display a lack of confidence).

➤ *Never, ever, ever, simply read out what is on a slide.* It is extremely patronising to the audience, adds no value at all and wastes time. Of course you will be amplifying the contents of a slide and will inevitably be using some of the same words but please do not read verbatim.

➤ When it is *time for questions*, put your notes down, blank the screen (press B or W), do not start packing your briefcase and give the audience your complete attention. A good tactic in smaller rooms is to sit for questions as it seems to change the dynamic of the session and leads to more balanced discussion. By blanking the screen rather than shutting the system down, you can get back to a key slide if it helps with answering the question. If you can answer the question do so succinctly and then check if you have answered their query.

If it has not, have one more go but avoid getting into a protracted dialogue with one person as this bores the audience and can lead to increasing defensiveness. After two attempts, politely suggest that you and that person continue the discussion afterwards. If you cannot answer the question, say so and commit publicly to finding out and getting back to the person as soon as possible. Never bluff. Chances are someone in the audience *does* know the answer and your hard-won credibility can be destroyed in an instant when they catch you out. One tactic to help avoid that is to reflect the question back to the audience and ask if anyone else can offer advice.

➤ *Remember why you are there in the first place.* If it is to get approval or permission, funding or senior support, do not leave without either securing that agreement or finding out what will happen next. Too many presenters, in their haste to leave the scene, end up not really being sure what was agreed. Of course this may suit some audiences and management teams who may be quite happy with 'no decision'. Keep it professional but do not let the group off the hook. Saying 'So, ladies and gentlemen, do I have your agreement to proceed?' will leave no one in any doubt that you were there for a reason and will normally prompt the chair of the meeting to intervene.

➤ Finally, do not forget to *review your performance.* If it went well, take a few minutes to 're-run the tape' and spot the key moments. Was it your preparation? Which slide really seemed to grab their attention? Was finishing early significant? Similarly, if you feel it could be improved, how? Did you not start confidently? Were there too many slides? Was the structure not clear? Or perhaps one question caught you out. Use the review information to consolidate or change your practice. Do not simply breathe a sigh of relief that it is over and rush back to something more familiar. If presenting in tandem with others, agree beforehand to keep an eye on the other person's performance and provide mutual feedback afterwards.

To summarise briefly, making presentations is a perfectly normal management activity. People do them every day and they are still alive! However, like any management practice, there are some key principles to learn and follow, and some quite simple tactics to sharpen up your approach. A good presentation can significantly improve the chances of influencing a team or meeting. It can improve your personal visibility and credibility within your organisation and most groups will be grateful that you took the time to be professional. However, if your case or proposal is poor, no amount of slick presentation will save it. Therefore, ensure that the purpose and robustness of your case is clear before starting to plan how to deliver it on the day.

CHAPTER 7

Effective management reports

Quite simply, a management report is a way of providing people with the information they need to make decisions. You may hear on the news that some organisation or another has issued a report. Sometimes these follow problems or crises, on other occasions they are written to change opinion or herald a new way of working. Whatever their origin, they have just the one real purpose – to influence decision-making, either by the direct recipient or by later readers.

Some reports are many hundreds of pages long, others may be two pages or less. Ultimately the length will depend on the:

➤ topic
➤ depth of analysis required
➤ conventions of the organisation concerned
➤ likely readership of the final document.

However, underneath all the differences in size, content, style and imagery, there are some common principles.

Reports should be simple, clear and as brief as possible. If you can write reports effectively you will promote clarity and speed in decision-making, and enhance your reputation. This short section offers advice on the process you need to follow in order to write an effective business report. It is important to note that writing concisely does take time and effort.

> One writer once apologised for the length of one of his letters, regretting that he 'did not have the time to write a shorter one'.
>
> Blaise Pascal, *Lettres Provinciales* (1656–1657), no. 16.

The process of sifting through all the information that *could* be included and settling on what *must* be included will help with the clarity of your message and is worth the time involved.

STEP 1: DEFINE THE PURPOSE

Make sure you are clear about why you are writing the report, what should be included and who your readers are. Vagueness about purpose will lead to an unsuitable report. Make sure a written report is what is needed. For some purposes an oral report or a presentation would be better. If in doubt ask the main recipient(s) before starting the work.

Before saying yes to any request to prepare a report, your questions must include:

➤ What is the report intended to achieve?

➤ Who will be receiving/reading/acting on the report?

➤ What is the scope (data/timescales/subject matter)?

➤ When is it required?

➤ What amount of detail is required?

➤ Are there any constraints/non-negotiables/no-go areas I need to be aware of before I start?

Two personal examples will illustrate the need to ask these questions rather than make assumptions.

AS: I once had a report sent back to me from a public sector client for more work. The advice was that the report was 'too short'. This might sound bizarre in a world that values brevity and economy of effort but further investigation provided the answer. The report was now going to be used by a large number of senior public officials to influence future social policy and so it needed to have more explicit data and analysis to justify the fundamental change of approach being proposed. In short the original document lacked 'gravitas' and needed to have its authority strengthened. For this particular client this included the report's physical size.

AP: I worked with a private sector client for whom I had carried out some research and staff interviews. Armed with the results I asked the client what sort of report they needed. Their response was 'we don't want a report – we're paying you to know your stuff, not charge us for writing it down. Just come along to our next meeting and give a short presentation with your advice on what we should do next!'

In both cases, the client was right, and it is first and foremost the client's needs that have to be met. You may enjoy preparing a technically faultless treatise on your pet topic, but unless it helps the reader to make a decision it is just wasted effort.

An example of a clear purpose (with our emphases) is:

'A report for the *Directorate Manager, Support Services* on the *sickness absence* of all *directly employed catering staff* during financial year *2010/11*, identifying the *main factors* and *making recommendations* for *reducing absence*'

This may look quite wordy, and will certainly not win the Booker Prize, but it is unambiguous, with a precise topic and scope, an intended readership, and a clear purpose.

STEP 2: INVESTIGATE THE TOPIC

This depends on the subject and purpose of the report. Your aim should be to gather enough information to enable good decisions to be made. This may include:

➤ qualitative (e.g. the views of staff) and quantitative (e.g. £s spent) information
➤ information from inside the organisation
➤ comparative information from other organisations or industries
➤ information from books or professional journals
➤ information gathered using questionnaires, focus groups or interviews.

STEP 3: ORGANISE YOUR INFORMATION

Having explored the topic, you will need to organise your information and your thoughts in a way that makes it easy to turn them into a report. One way of doing this is to write down all the ideas, issues, thoughts and facts you have gathered onto one large sheet of paper. You can then begin to group or link together the issues. Mind-mapping is another useful technique. (A Google search on 'Tony Buzan' will provide more information on this approach.)

Keep asking yourself, *'What are my readers looking for and what is the best way to sort this information to meet those needs?'*

STEP 4: STRUCTURE YOUR REPORT

A typical structure would be as follows.

➤ Title, author, date clearly stated at the top of the first page. Placing an abbreviated form of this information in a footer section on each page can help ensure that if some pages become detached the context is not lost.
➤ Contents and page numbers (only required for lengthy reports, say 10+ pages).
➤ Executive summary, which summarises the purpose of the report, highlights its main findings and alerts readers to the critical recommendations. (Executive

summaries are particularly useful for long or complex reports, or reports where there is an expectation of you getting to the critical point quickly). Remember that some people will only read the executive summary so it needs to be concise but completely clear. If your report is very short, this section can be merged with your introduction.

➤ Introduction, which details the purpose of the report, your method of working and the main sources of information you used.

➤ Background, which puts the report in context, gives a short explanation of how the topic came to be of such importance, includes any relevant history and provides a cross reference to any similar work being carried out elsewhere.

➤ Discussion, which is the main body of the report. It tells the readers the main facts and issues, their possible implications and the options available.

➤ Summary and conclusions, which restate the purpose of the report and give your conclusions. In long reports, a slimmed down version of this section is inserted before the discussion and is called the executive summary.

➤ Recommendations, which states what you think should be done in future, not forgetting to cover the detailed implementation plan and any consequences that should be taken into account.

➤ Appendix, which is for material only needed by those studying the report in depth. If charts or tables are highly relevant they should be included in the discussion section.

Note that in a very short report you might be able to leave out or combine sections.

STEP 5: CHECK AND REVISE

Always read through your report and check for spelling and grammatical errors. Even better, ask a couple of people who are not experts in your area to read it for you. Ask these questions:

➤ Does it meet its intended purpose?

➤ Is it clear, simple and persuasive?

➤ Is it easily readable and presented in a logical order?

➤ Is it the length it is because it needs to be, or because I haven't been concise/ thorough enough?

USE OF DRAFT REPORTS

If you are genuinely not sure you have covered exactly what is required and want to get the reader(s) involved in shaping the final version – in terms of its main message or content – it can be useful to publish a first draft and circulate this, asking for comments. This technique is not to be used as a way of getting the reader to do your job for you, nor should the draft be so thin and disjointed that it lacks any credibility. However, in an era where inclusivity and participation are positive management approaches, asking others to comment on a draft and suggest minor changes can sometimes make the difference between ownership and rejection. Do not use this technique if you are under severe time pressures as it can slow the process down, particularly if there are a lot of people to contact.

Also do not consult unless you are genuinely interested in, and prepared to accept, the responses you will get. Consultation exercises, particularly in the public sector, are often perceived as being somewhat shallow exercises where only one option is published for comment, and the decision is widely rumoured to have been made already. Make sure that the time and effort you are asking respondents to commit to the process is worthwhile or you will lose their future interest.

AND FINALLY . . .

If your organisation has a house style for fonts, page layout, logos, images, etc. use it. Otherwise, you should avoid fancy fonts or frequent use of italic, coloured or bold text. Cursive handwriting may work in the family Christmas letter but looks unprofessional in a report and can be hard to read. Left-justified 10- or 12-point Arial, Helvetica or Times fonts provide easily readable text.

Converting your report to PDF format prior to its circulation can ensure that it remains in its original form and is not re-edited without your knowledge. However, be aware that, despite their claims, some computer operating systems can struggle to display this format successfully so it is always a good idea to ask all recipients to acknowledge safe receipt and legibility, especially if circulating your report by email.

CHAPTER 8

Over to you

If you have got this far you will have realised that good people management is not *complicated* but it is *complex*. It does not require massive intellect, nor does it have to have a complete set of manuals for every situation. For you to be an effective people manager we suggest that you need the following.

➤ A willingness to start by placing trust in people (the same trust you would like your employer to place in you).

➤ A belief that your staff want to do a good job and, given the right environment and support, will give their best.

➤ A genuine interest in what motivates and interests your staff.

➤ A desire to spend time giving and receiving feedback.

➤ A recognition of the need to be 'relentlessly reasonable' and to persevere even when the initial response to that reasonableness is not what you expected.

➤ The flexibility to adopt different approaches based on the needs of the situation and the member of staff concerned.

In other words, good people management is all about *character*. You don't need to be a genius to do it well, but you will need determination, self-awareness and resilience.

Unlike the process of acquiring technical knowledge, where one fact or approach adds to existing material, learning about management can often challenge prior assumptions and practice. This can be uncomfortable and those people who prefer not to live with the struggle and ambiguity may simply put this book down and go back to their old ways. We strongly believe that there is no learning without change and no useful change without learning. Therefore the only significant purpose of this book is to bring about a change in practice.

There are many models used to describe the learning and change process. One that has stood the test of time is David Kolb's Learning Cycle. It looks like this.

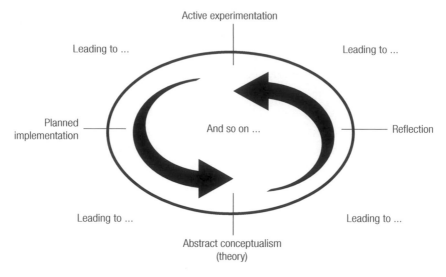

FIGURE 9.1 Kolb's Learning Cycle

Kolb argues that, whilst the cycle can be entered at any point, learning tends to start with an *experience* or activity. This may be positive or negative, affirming or challenging, but the point is that something *experiential* triggers the learning process.

Following that initial experience is a period of *reflection*. This may be short or long for different people but it is a process where the learner muses on what has happened and how close or far away it is to their expectations and prior beliefs. For many people this is the most challenging phase as it is where most of the struggle and ambiguity lies, and there are two ways forward.

1 The first is to simply reject the new experience as being so different from those prior beliefs that it must be wrong (and so return to the old ways).
2 The second is to use that struggle to challenge and test existing practice and accept the possibility that other approaches are worthy of further consideration.

The first of these is often referred to as the 'flight or fight' response. We occasionally come across clients who find our employee-led alternatives to top-down authoritative management so unsettling (cue images of out of control staff, chaos and mayhem), that they switch off or leave (flight), or try desperately to create scenarios that our alternative approach would fail to tackle (fight). In both cases the mental energy that might have been used to seriously weigh up the material and then come to a considered view is simply used up by these other behaviours. The inevitable result is that learning stops immediately and pre-emptive blame takes its place. You will recall that earlier we suggested that you can either blame or you can learn but you can't do both at the same time!

For those who stay with the struggle, Kolb's model then suggests that the reflection stage gives way to developing new *theories and models* to explain the new experience. At this point, assuming the person has accepted that other approaches may be useful, this is the process whereby they (in theory) 'find a home' for the learning alongside existing ideas, for later use.

The fourth part of Kolb's cycle involves the process of *planning and implementing* the new thinking, an activity that helps with the consolidation of the learning as the person rehearses their thoughts and then puts them into practice.

Given the cyclical nature of the model, that implementation provokes a new experience and the process repeats itself.

As with all models, including the ones we have offered in this book, its simplicity is its Achilles' heel. Not all learning follows that neat pattern; some people prefer one or two of the activities over the others and will therefore pay less attention to some parts of the cycle, and some organisations value action over thinking so much that there is no incentive to engage in such a cerebral process. Sometimes we condition ourselves to devalue the reflective process, or perhaps we don't have time for it.

> Imagine you were in your office (assuming you have one), staring into space, perhaps with your feet on the desk, thinking through an issue or just reflecting on an event. Your boss arrives at the door and catches you in 'mid-thought'. Most of us would hastily adopt a more professional position, not just out of courtesy, but also in order to demonstrate busyness. It seems that in many walks of life, being busy is preferred to being effective!

Despite these caveats, the model can still help us understand where our learning may be 'out of balance' and can alert us to the risks of 'running away' when we encounter learning that challenges our current practice.

FIVE CHALLENGES

As you prepare to close this book, hopefully not for the last time, we would like to suggest five simple and effective ways of maintaining the management learning journey. They cost little or no money; some require some time and effort, but together they place you unashamedly in charge of your future development.

1 **Seek feedback on how you are doing as a manager.**
   There is no need to create elaborate mechanisms to do this; simply take every opportunity to get feedback from those around you. If the feedback is good, be proud. If it suggests improvements are needed, better to find out early. Of course if, on reflection, you simply cannot agree with the feedback you are free to carry

on as before but at least that will be an informed decision. Some organisations engage in 360° appraisal schemes and these can be highly beneficial. However, you don't have wait for the formal scheme. Ask some of the people you trust 'How am I doing?', and then do something with the feedback you get. If you don't act on it then don't expect people to give honest and helpful answers the next time you ask!

2 **Find a mentor.**
Mentors are people whose wisdom and perspective you trust but who do not manage you nor do they have any significant influence on your day-to-day work. Typically they will be senior figures in your organisation, or another enterprise, who agree to meet with you periodically to challenge your thinking, give you new insights and encourage you in your development. If you find the right someone for you, be sure to use their time sparingly and wisely, and have a clear purpose and outcome for each session. Most people are flattered to be asked to mentor someone but their patience will be sorely tested if all you want is an idle chat with them every so often.

3 **Shadow those who do what you would like to do!**
If you spot people who just seem naturally able to tackle issues in a way you would like to, regardless of their relative status, why not ask them if you could accompany them the next time they do it, so that you can learn direct? That is one form of shadowing. The second is where you spend a block of time with a key figure (say a day or a week) in order to get a full appreciation of their job, the context and their challenges. Again this takes time rather than money and most people would be flattered to be asked. As with mentoring, make sure both of you understand the purpose of the arrangement and please get the support of your immediate colleagues, particularly if you do the second form of shadowing, as they will have to cover your absence.

4 **Develop and update a personal development plan (PDP).**
Chapter 2 outlines a simple but powerful approach to creating the sort of personal development plan that recognises the whole person. Some people like plans, others find them restrictive, but most people agree that the *process of planning* is useful and can create the momentum for change. However you choose to do it, articulating your priorities and goals, asking how well you are doing in pursuit of these and then committing yourself to some action as a result, can act as a catalyst for your continuing development.

One of the most useful things about a personal development plan is that it is yours! No one has to see it, it does not need to be set out in long sentences, or neat boxes. In fact it does not have to make sense to anyone else at all. As long as it helps you, it is perfectly designed.

5   **Become a reflective practitioner.**
This is not the place to rehearse all the theory and practice on this subject but it is enough to say that effective practitioners tend to be those who constantly monitor what they do (both in the moment and afterwards), who see any setbacks and challenges as valuable sources of learning and who are not afraid to try new approaches. They accept the principle that 'all change starts with me' and they tend to look at their own practice first rather than looking for someone or something else to blame.

CONCLUSION

We conclude as we started. Management is a noble and important profession, and managing people is one of the most important activities within any organisation. Our hope is that, if you are new to this field, this book has given you the tools and insights you need to step into the people-management role confidently and competently. If you have been a manager for some years, we hope that the book has affirmed and enhanced your current practice. If it has challenged that practice, we wish you well in the struggle.

Being well managed at work should not be a bonus, something to be treasured on the rare occasions it happens. It should be the norm. People who are well managed and supported tend to give of their best. Those who are not tend to leave! Some leave physically and find new jobs. Others simply switch off mentally; they do the minimum required, keep their heads down and go home complaining about their employer.

It is estimated that the total cost of losing someone, recruiting a replacement and getting them up to speed is at least 20% of the annual salary for that post. Lets be clear – this means that for someone who is paid £20 000pa, their leaving will cost their employer at least £4 000. If people leave for career advancement and create the space for new talent to blossom then all well and good. If they leave due to poor people management that is an expensive 'own goal' by the organisation.

Therefore good people management affects the bottom line of any enterprise. Whether that is profit, restoring health, good government, services provided or money saved, the impact of poor people management is damaging to the organisation and its ability to operate effectively in the future. Therefore looking after your people will be one of the most important contributions you will make in your career.

We wish you well in your practice, and welcome to the world of good people management!

If you wish to continue your learning dialogue with us, or have comments about the book, please feel free to contact either of us via www.developmentconsultancy. co.uk

Selected reading list

This is a practical book and we have deliberately kept to a minimum the number of theories about management we mention. However, our actions as managers are deeply affected by what we think about people, organisations, work and many other issues. Therefore we offer this short reading list not as a way of gathering theory for its own sake, but as a way for you to challenge and develop your working theories of management.

Effective People (2nd ed.) by Stephen Prosser (Oxford: Radcliffe Publishing; 2010). Specifically aimed at NHS managers who want to improve their practice.

Leadership is an Art by Max DePree (London: Currency; 2004). Short, highly readable and full of profound values.

Maverick by Ricardo Semler (London: Arrow; 1994). The story of an unconventional but successful approach to running an organisation.

The Fifth Discipline by Peter Senge (New York: Random House; 2010). A real classic. Goes beyond simplistic solutions and explores how and why people and organisations learn, or fail to learn.

The Future of Management by Gary Hamel (Boston: Harvard Business School Press; 2007). An erudite and provocative argument for why we need to change the way organisations are managed.

Understanding Organisations by Charles Handy (London: Penguin; 1993). Easy to read, lucid and wide-ranging. A good introduction to management and organisations.

Index